A Child By
Any Means

A Child By Any Means

MODERN TREATMENTS FOR INFERTILITY
AND THE ISSUES THEY RAISE

MAGGIE JONES

PIATKUS

© 1989 Maggie Jones
First published in 1989 by Judy Piatkus
(Publishers) Limited, 5 Windmill Street,
London W1P 1HF

British Library Cataloguing in Publication Data

Jones, Maggie, *1953* –
  A child by any means.
  1. Man. Infertility
  I. Title
  616.6'92

  ISBN 0 – 86188 – 830 – 8

Edited by Maggie Daykin
Designed by Sue Ryall

Typeset by Action Typesetting Limited, Gloucester
Printed and bound in Great Britain by
Mackays of Chatham PLC

Contents

Acknowledgements

We would like to thank Professor R. G. Edwards for granting us permission to reproduce the diagram on page 22 from the book *Conception in the Human Female* published by Academic Press, and Thorsons Publishing Group Limited for the diagram on page 16 from the book *Now or Never* by Bostock and Jones, 1987.

Introduction

Many books have been published on the subject of infertility, the new techniques which may overcome it, and the ethical issues involved, but none have looked closely into how the couples concerned feel, what solutions they have come to, or how they feel towards the children born as a result of new technology, especially those who are not their genetic offspring. There are further questions too. Why do most people want children? What are the problems faced by the infertile? What are the new options available to them? How do they feel about these options? How will they adapt to a new kind of parenthood? What are children born through IVF, through embryo, sperm and egg donation, going to feel? What can be done to protect their interests? What rights do they have to learn about their origins and about their biological parents? Will the new technologies give birth to families that are no different to conventional ones or will we be creating new kinds of stepfamilies, with the sort of problems many of these now face?

Sometimes this book may appear to raise more questions than answers, because I believe the best decisions about new fertility treatment will only come through listening to the voices of those who have experienced it or are affected by it – or will be in the future – the infertile, their families, and the children they may ultimately be helped to bear.

Whether you are 'infertile' and, in trying to conceive, need information on all the options and implications, or simply want to be better informed on this major – many would say 'vital' – issue of our time, I hope this book will be a helpful introduction to these complex issues.

MIRACLES OF MODERN SCIENCE

Through the various combinations of techniques for obtaining eggs and sperm and for fertilising and reimplanting them, there are now at least 16 different ways to have a child.

- A child can be conceived naturally or through artificial insemination or through in vitro fertilisation (IVF).
- The eggs can come from the mother or from a donor, the sperm from the father or a donor, or both can come from a donor.
- The baby can be carried in the womb of a surrogate mother, who also provided the egg, or a host mother, who carries a child which is not genetically hers.
- A child can also be conceived posthumously through frozen eggs, sperm or embryos.

A chart detailing these various combinations appears in Chapter 4, where the techniques are fully explained. These new scientific techniques which have enabled infertile couples to achieve their dream have brought with them a host of other developments that a few years ago would have been dismissed as science fiction but have now become reality:

- A grandmother bore and gave birth to her daughter's triplets.
- Twin embryos were stored deep frozen for months and then born 18 months apart.
- Babies born prematurely at 22 weeks have survived, some without handicap.
- Women who have passed the menopause are being helped to conceive and give birth.

Indeed, science has moved so fast that medical opinion, popular opinion and the law have not been able to keep pace, giving rise to practical, social, emotional and ethical problems.

REACTIONS

In July 1982, following worldwide debate and concern at what was happening in the wake of the first successful attempt at in vitro fertilisation (IVF), the 'test-tube baby' treatment, the British government set up a committee, headed by Dame Mary Warnock, to look into the questions of human fertilisation and embryology, and other aspects of treatment for the infertile. The subsequent report, published in July 1984, provided a basis for legislation and, after further wide consultation the government published its White Paper on Human Fertilisation and Embryology, in December 1987. This was in the very same month that the European Parliament considered reproductive technologies.

The British Government's proposed legislation, as outlined

> **The Warnock report concluded that** *certain infertility treatments such as IVF and those involving donated eggs, sperm and embryos should be permitted, subject to statutory control by an independent body. The report also made recommendations on surrogate motherhood (commercial surrogacy should be made illegal and surrogacy was to be discouraged), the storage and disposal of human embryos, eggs and sperm, the status of children born after embryos, egg or sperm donation and the development of infertility services generally, including counselling.*
>
> *Warnock recommended that a Statutory Licensing Authority be set up to inspect and control centres in which the new infertility treatments and embryo research might be carried out. This Authority should be 'independent of Government, health authorities and research institutions' and not made up entirely by doctors and similar professionals. In 1985 the Royal College of Obstetricians and Gynaecologists and the Medical Research Council set up a Voluntary Licensing Authority (VLA) along these lines to act as a watchdog in the meantime. Centres working with the new fertility treatments were invited to apply for approval and licence. So far all centres have done so, and despite some disagreements have abided by the VLA's decisions.*

in the White Paper, will finally ensure that children born in the UK following the donation of sperm, eggs or embryos will be the legitimate children of the family into which they are born. (For too long such children have been technically illegitimate.) It is also proposed that the Statutory Licensing Authority will hold information on donors, including the name and date of birth of the child and a reference number for the donor. It is suggested that all adults over the age of 18 should have a legal right to find out whether they were born by egg, sperm or embryo donation and if so, have access to non-identifying information about the donor.

However, the White Paper did not reply to the question of whether non-commercial surrogacy should be made legal and be provided by infertility centres with appropriate selection of surrogate mothers, couples and counselling. Consequently, doctors are not sure whether they might be breaking the law in helping to arrange surrogate pregnancies in limited circumstances, as some believe they should. Indeed, this is a dilemma on an international scale.

In Australia, the committees which considered aspects of assisted reproduction stopped short of recommending the actual criminalisaton of surrogate motherhood, feeling that if surrogate contracts were not recognised in law and advertising to recruit surrogate mothers were illegal this would be enough to discourage it. Only in Canada did the Ontario Law Reform Commission suggest that surrogate contracts be recognised, and be made enforceable, even if this meant seizing the child from the surrogate mother. The Commission felt that this would be in the best interests of the child, and that the surrogate mother would know the score in advance. However, this has not passed into law.

LEADING ISSUES

One of the most emotive issues to be raised universally following the development of IVF is the question of the rights of the embryos created outside the human body and using such embryos for research:

- Should surplus embryos created be destroyed?
- Should they be frozen for future use by the couple concerned?
- If not in the end wanted, should they be donated to someone else? Or should they be used for research?
- At what stage does the embryo become a human being?
- Can embryos be used for research and if so, up to what stage in their development?

Some doctors and scientists argue that it is a pity that embryo research has become so closely linked with the provision of infertility treatments, many of which are not actually affected by it.

Those who have personally suffered the tragic human consequences of being unable to have a child strongly protest their right to attempt to overcome their infertility with the new techniques available. Indeed, not only the majority of people who have experienced problems in conceiving, but also the majority of the general public, would support most forms of assisted reproduction, but there is fundamental opposition to either the principle or the various techniques available. The main arguments against assisted reproduction are:

- **That it is not natural.** People who support this view often say that it is not right to over-ride God or nature in this matter, that a couple or individual should be reconciled to their childlessness and find other ways of fulfilment. The counter argument is that most modern medical treatment could be viewed as 'unnatural' and that to reject it as such is falling into the extremism showed by religious groups such as Christian Scientists and Jehovah's Witnesses who will not even allow a dying relative a blood transfusion.
- **That infertility is not a disease.** Though infertility may not strictly be a disease, it is often the result of a disease, such as diabetes or a sexually transmitted infection in the man, or a pelvic infection, past pelvic surgery, endometriosis or disease of the ovaries in a woman. The problem may be a malfunction of the hormonal system which, if not considered a disease, must be a disorder. Infertility is a fundamental malfunctioning of the human body and as such deserves medical treatment.
- **Having children is a luxury.** This argument is that even

if infertility is a disease or disorder, it does not actually threaten the sufferer's life or continued existence, and therefore is not a priority for treatment. Having children is considered to be a luxury rather than to be an essential part of living.

The opposite view is that reproducing himself is biologically the main purpose of man's existence. Illnesses which occur in later life, when a man has had his children, are unimportant in biological terms because they do not affect his ability to reproduce himself. Therefore it could be argued that they are less, not more, deserving of treatment.

- **Infertility treatment involves unacceptable practices.** Some argue that while straightforward treatments of infertility, such as repairing diseased tubes or giving drugs which do not have harmful side-effects might be acceptable, treatments which involve the donation or storing of sperm, eggs and embryos or which call for the participation of third parties such as surrogate mothers are not.

  The Catholic Church also argues that procedures involving collection of sperm by masturbation are unacceptable. *Humanae Vitae,* Pope Paul VI's famous encyclical, issued in 1968, came out against the use of 'artificial' birth control methods by practising Catholics, and said quite clearly that the Church would not permit the separation or exclusion of the 'procreative intention or of the conjugal relationship.' Previously Pius XII wrote: 'To reduce the shared life of a married couple and the act of married love to a mere organic activity for transmitting semen would be like turning the domestic home, the sanctuary of the family, into a biological laboratory.' This view clearly expresses the disquiet which many Catholics, and others, feel about assisted reproduction. More recently, the Catholic Church has reiterated its opposition to IVF and other new reproductive techniques. Against this view, many argue that masturbation is a natural sexual outlet and if the child is born of a loving relationship, masturbation for the purpose of creating a child cannot be wrong.

- **Many treatments involve 'genealogical bewilderment' for the child.** This is one of the strongest arguments against techniques which separate genetic and social parenthood.

However, for centuries children have been adopted, brought up by step-parents and conceived outside wedlock, and rising divorce and remarriage rates mean that an increasing number of children live with one parent who is not their natural parent and step- or half-brothers and sisters. Children conceived through assisted reproduction techniques and having different genetic and social parents would probably not add greatly to those numbers.

Whether it is fair to specifically create children for such a situation is more difficult to answer although the evidence from children born through artificial insemination by donor is that while it might cause them some problems, few would prefer not to exist.

- **Why put such effort into creating a child when many children still wait to be adopted?** This is a valid question but, as fully discussed in Chapter 1 many people do want their own child – or a child as close to being their own as possible – and many women want to experience pregnancy, childbirth and breastfeeding. Also, many people are not considered suitable to adopt because of their age, previous divorce, race or other factors over which they have no control. Others do not feel able to cope with the demands made by children who may have had past unhappy experiences or who have severe disabilities. Others may not pass adoption screening procedures for reasons which are never divulged to them … often it may simply be that the social workers who assessed the couple do not like them or consider they would not make suitable parents for reasons which may be hard to qualify.

  Most people adopt because they are unable to have their own children, not because they specifically want to bring up other children. It seems reasonable that many people might want to try every possibility of having a child which is their own, or at least of their partner's before thinking of adoption.

- **Assisted reproduction inevitably results in some experimentation on embryos.** Some assisted reproduction treatments such as IVF will involve the sacrifice of some embryos which cannot be used for implantation either because they seem to be developing less well than others, or because too many embryos have grown successfully. Embryos also have to be examined to check that they are normal and this could be considered as 'experimentation'. For those who find the concept of experimenting on embryos abhorrent, IVF and many other treatments will not be acceptable.

Those without a voice in these many and varied debates are the children who are yet to be born. In the meantime, the children who have already been brought up by non-genetic parents through adoption, divorce and remarriage and AID have many lessons to teach us. We shall be looking at this aspect in Chapter 7.

A CHILD
BY ANY MEANS

1
Why we want children

In recent years the number of articles on couples' struggles to overcome their infertility have grown apace. More than ever, it seems, we want to have children. After a brief period in the 1960s and 70s when a vocal minority of couples sought freedom from the ties and responsibilities of family life, and stated concern about the future of our overpopulated planet, the family is back in fashion. Not only do some politicians sing the virtues of the family unit, not always for altruistic reasons, but we are seeing a new interest in children as part of our consumer culture, with the growth of designer toys, baby equipment and babywear. Even Hollywood epics have given the star role to baby.

Why do so many of us want children so much? Is it the age-old biological instinct which prevails? Or is a baby just another desirable possession – like a house, car, new kitchen – even the ultimate status symbol?

Those who *don't* want children – at least not until they have achieved all their other goals – often see motherhood as so low in status and children so demanding and disrupting to an ordered lifestyle that they fail to understand what reasons there could be for wanting children. So, there is a dual attitude to motherhood: on the one hand it is seen in a romantic way as a woman's vocation and true role in life, and on the other as a boring, repetitive task peripheral to career success or social advancement. Reluctance to take on such a commitment may

1

also be influenced by the fact that so many marriages break down, that there are many unwanted pregnancies (the Family Planning Association estimates 200,000 a year), and that physical and sexual child abuse is rising. Such considerations tend to blind some people to the hope, joys and pleasures also involved in having children – the thrill and fascination of watching them grow and develop and the wonderful relationship of love and intimacy which parents can and do discover with their children.

In particular, some people may find it hard to understand the desperation of those who find themselves unable to have children, and wonder why they are prepared, with or without the help of new medical technology, to go to extraordinary lengths to have a child they can call their own. They may even perceive the infertile as selfish, or neurotic people, who should accept their situation and make the best of it, or even be grateful that they are not burdened with children and can be 'childfree'.

Yet this question of wanting or not wanting children is a very recent one. Only in the present century has there been any real choice for the great majority of people.

THE OLD FAMILY ORDER

In the past, sexual liaisons led almost inevitably to the birth of children and social structures were created to prevent sexual relationships outside of a stable marriage bond, and to guarantee that the children a man brought up were his. Any children born to the marriage were assumed to be the genetic descendents of their parents, the children of their own flesh and blood. When relationships did occur outside of marriage, the children of such unions were branded illegitimate and did not enjoy the rights of children conceived within a marriage.

THE FAMILY TODAY

Even today, when Western societies accept the idea of an equal marriage partnership, children are still considered for the most part the property of their parents, who can control almost every aspect of their lives. Only under extreme circumstances, when their life or safety is held to be at stake, can children be removed from their parents or extended families and taken into care.

Children of a marriage are still assumed to be the genetic offspring of their parents, and if they are not, it is often kept secret. As recounted in myth and literature from earliest times, where a child is not the blood relation of both parents, there may be trouble: stepchildren persecuted by stepmothers or stepfathers, a changeling taking the place of a couple's natural child and causing problems in the family, adopted children who turn out badly in one way or another. These stories, buried deep in our consciousness, continue to influence our ideas and create the feeling that only our own biological or blood children will truly satisfy us.

Parents and grandparents are delighted when their children or grandchildren inherit clearly recognisable characteristics from them. It gives them a sense of immortality – that something of them is going on into the future and will endure after their death. In having children we fulfil our biological purpose, and although few people today would say this was the most important reason for their existence, at some deep level there still seems a recognition that this is the case.

In many societies adoption has always existed to care for orphaned children and to provide offspring for those unable to have their own. Adoption is normally recognised through a formal declaration that this child will be treated 'as if' he or she were the natural child of the family, whether this is recognised in law or not. However, some family members can not forget the absence of the blood tie, and the child may be made very aware of this, or have to prove his gratitude and loyalty over the years.

DEVELOPMENT OF CONTRACEPTION

In modern times family foundations have been rocked by a rapid series of changes, all based on the development of tech-

nologies which, for the first time in human history, enable men
and women to effectively separate sexual experience from
reproduction. The first major breakthrough was the development of modern methods of contraception – although contraception has existed in various forms for centuries. These were
mainly spermicidal preparations inserted into the woman's
vagina – pessaries made out of crocodile-dung were reported
in ancient Egypt – or condoms such as those made of sheep's
gut popularised by Casanova in the eighteenth century. In the
nineteenth century the use of home-made vaginal sponges and
withdrawal were recommended, and by the end of the century
early caps to cover the cervix and spermicidal pessaries were
developed.

However, these contraceptives were not very effective, not
widely available and, indeed, not socially approved of. Condoms were used more to prevent the passing on of sexually
transmitted diseases than to prevent pregnancies. Only in the
mid-twentieth century were more effective contraceptive
methods made available to ordinary men and women.

THE SEXUAL REVOLUTION

In the early 1960s came the real breakthroughs: the contraceptive Pill, IUDs suitable for childless women, and quick, safe
methods of both male and female sterilisation. These much
safer methods of contraception revolutionised social attitudes
towards sex and its expression. The 'permissive society' made
possible sexual relationships with no commitment on either
side to form a permanent liaison and have a family. By the late
1960s abortion had been made legal on both medical and social
grounds, divorce law was reformed to enable couples to split up
more easily and remove the concept of 'guilty' and 'innocent'
parties and family planning clinics had opened their doors to
unmarried people seeking contraceptive advice and supplies.

The sexual revolution was on the whole greeted as not a bad
thing, freeing men and women to find greater happiness,
greater sexual fulfilment and, for women especially, making it
possible to compete on more equal terms with men in the

workplace and exercise personal control over whether or when to have children.

However, this new freedom was not without its dark side. Many women found that without the protection of marriage and the threat of pregnancy, men used them for sexual fulfilment without providing the security they needed for a happy relationship. Even 'effective' contraception was not without its side-effects and risks – which the woman usually had to bear – and there were occasions when it failed and an unwanted pregnancy resulted. Few women have an abortion without considerable feelings of sadness and guilt and many underwent the experience without the support of their partner who had entered the relationship with no intention of a lasting commitment.

THE NEW WOMAN

Perhaps the most significant effect of the separation of sexuality from reproduction has been the freeing of many women from purely domestic responsibilities. During the two world wars women proved that they could work outside the home and the numbers of women in employment outside the home has increased steadily. Women have also achieved higher and higher offices. The numbers of women doctors, politicians, lawyers and executives continue to rise, though many say too slowly.

However, pressures are still brought to bear on women through laws, religion and social structures which assume that women will give birth to the children on whom society depends, and take the central role in bringing them up. Because it is assumed that women will have children, some employers are still reluctant to take women on. Also, although most working women now have the statutory right to paid maternity leave, it is not unusual for firms to pass them over for promotion or in other ways curtail their career after they have had a baby. In particular, women who can no longer work some shifts or stay late at the office because they have a young family may find it difficult to get promotion or well-paid jobs. This may discourage some ambitious women from having families, but it probably also makes more women give up work to become full-time mothers because such pressures make it not worth trying to succeed at both. A large number of women, however, do not really have a choice; financial necessity obliges them to take whatever work they can find.

For these various reasons family size has continued to fall, and there has been an increasing trend for many women to delay childbearing and have fewer children later in life. In the UK, the number of first babies born to mothers who have been married for between 10 and 14 years has doubled over the last ten years, and births to mothers aged 30 to 39 had increased from nearly 112,000 in 1974 out of 640,000 live births to 165,500 out of 637,000 live births in 1984.

As women in many countries have become less financially dependent on their husbands and have found alternative sources of satisfaction to being simply wives and mothers, divorce rates also have soared. One in three marriages is now expected to end in divorce. Remarriage is the norm, adding an increasing number of step-families and reconstituted families to the rising numbers of single-parent families left in the wake of divorce. These, together with dual-earning families with and without children, now outnumber the number of 'traditional' families with wage- or salary-earning father, stay-at-home mother and children. Also, as unemployment rises, increasing numbers of families have no wage-earner or have working wives and stay-at-home husbands.

HOMOSEXUALITY AND FAMILY LIFE

Along with changing attitudes to sexuality during the 1960s came a change in society's attitude to homosexuality. Legal reform meant that homosexual acts between consenting adults over 21 was no longer a crime, and increasing numbers of homosexual men and women chose to openly declare their sexual orientation and to live with their partner in a long-term relationship. Some men divorced their wives but kept up contact with their children; some lived with male partners *and* cared for the children of their previous marriage. Many lesbian women decided that they wanted to raise children, sometimes conceiving a child with a male friend sympathetic to their position or resorting to artificial insemination. Lesbian groups instructed women in 'self-insemination', a technique that has gone out of fashion since the AIDS epidemic started as many groups used homosexual men as sperm donors. Lesbian women may find a sympathetic doctor who will provide them with artificial insemination on the NHS or may be able to use a private clinic. (See also Chapter 4.)

TO HAVE OR HAVE NOT

As sexuality has been slowly and irresistibly separated from its consequence of producing children, many couples have increasingly given thought to whether they really want to have children or why they want to have children. The question, 'Why children?' is asked more and more today – indeed, it only has relevance now that such a choice, not to have children, is possible. There are many reasons why some find it hard to understand why most people choose to have children: for example, the expense, the disruption of careers and lifestyles, the exhaustion felt by many parents and the low status given to stay-at-home mothers. Some people also fear that their relationship with their partner will not only alter but actually suffer when children enter the picture. Women may also fear or simply wish to avoid the damage done to their bodies by pregnancy and childbirth in a culture which portrays only the very young and slim as being sexually desirable.

Even so, those who choose not to have children are still in a minority. Indeed, the separation of sexuality from reproduction may not be as complete as we like to think.

Many people find great difficulty in using contraception effectively, even if the consequences of having a baby are very undesirable. Studies have shown that a majority of young people do not use contraception the first time they have sexual intercourse and that a large number do not use effective contraception at all. This is not merely due to the difficulty in some countries or embarrassment of obtaining contraception, or even the conviction that 'It won't happen to me'. Many people have real difficulties in planning in a rational way for an irrational event. Others find the idea of risking pregnancy in itself exciting; or perhaps they would like a child, even if the circumstances are inappropriate.

Whatever the reasons, many pregnancies remain unplanned. The Family Planning Association estimates that there are about 200,000 unwanted pregnancies in Britain every year, over half of which end in abortion. The women who have unwanted pregnancies are no different from others. A study carried out in the United States by Kristen Luker, *Taking Chances: Abortion and the Decision Not to Contracept,* of young women who were having repeat abortions found that the only way in which these women differed from their peers was that they had been unlucky. However, theories that women who have repeat abortions have some underlying desire to get pregnant but then cannot go through with it may be true for a very few.

For many young people, the idea of pregnancy seems so horrific and so remote that they do not believe that it can happen to them. They certainly do not have sexual relationships out of an underlying need to have a baby.

Natural selection may have made sexuality pleasurable in order to lure the human race into reproducing itself, and most people – especially women – find babies and young children delightful and appealing, but they are also often afraid of them. The fact that in our society many people have never held a baby or seen one breastfed until they have their own makes most people afraid of handling infants because they do not know how to deal with them. In the small families of today, most people will have been too young to remember the birth of their younger brothers and sisters, and will have had no part in helping to bring them up.

The idea of having children seems frightening because most couples have no idea what to expect. So although parental instincts do exist, they seem to be outweighed today by fears of parental inadequacy. This has led to a proliferation of babycare books giving detailed information about how to change nappies, how to feed babies, how to bath them, dress them and help them sleep.

So is there such a thing as a 'maternal instinct'? It seems clear that women need to learn how to be mothers, whether from their own mothers, or from books and health professionals. Most aspects of motherhood do not come 'naturally', though the desire to do what is right for the baby does.

Mothers – and babies – have always been victims of medical and other advice, which has suggested such practices as not putting the baby to the breast till the milk comes in (this led to many maternal deaths from 'milk fever' in seventeenth century Europe); feeding on a four-hourly rota and leaving the baby to cry in between; bottle- rather than breastfeeding, or feeding the baby solid foods from an early age. Each generation of mothers has had to find her way through a mass of conflicting advice and misinformation; only the lucky ones, confident in their own instincts, have had the confidence to put such advice aside.

Some writers such as Elizabeth Badinter in her historical review, *The Myth of Motherhood*, have denied the existence of maternal instincts altogether, and found plenty of evidence to support this view, such as mothers who put their babies out to wet-nurses and showed no signs of grief when they died. However, other letters and books from this period show how much mothers did grieve their dead children and how much joy they found in the ones who thrived and grew. In every generation there will be a mixture of 'good' and 'bad' mothers. The support that society gives to mothers and families generally will have a lot to do with how well women cope with the pressures of motherhood.

REWARDS OF PARENTHOOD

Having children probably represents the most significant and traumatic experience a person ever experiences, apart from birth itself and death, neither of which we can have any memories of. In a way it forms the final separation from one's own childhood. People see themselves primarily as the children of their parents until, suddenly, they are parents in their turn.

Now they and their children are the immediate family. For the first time they are no longer expected to 'go home' for Christmas; home is now where the young children are.

In the immediate period after the birth, most parents find themselves the focus of praise and congratulations. Many mothers, in particular, find the few days after the birth an intensely rewarding time. They are made a tremendous fuss of by hospital staff, by relatives and friends, and by colleagues from work. If their working life has not given them any sense of reward and achievement, some mothers may even have more babies because they feel this is the only experience through which they have been acknowledged to have done something important.

Young, single women who get pregnant might have equally complex reasons for doing so. They may have had a child to 'trap a man into marriage', or to force parents and others to acknowledge a relationship, to fill up time if they and their partner are unemployed or unable to find worthwhile jobs, even to gain financial support or a home if local authorities give priority to single mothers or couples with children.

One young woman acknowledged that she had 'got herself pregnant' because it was proof to herself and her boyfriend that something important had happened between them. 'He said that just because we slept together didn't mean that the relationship was important to him. He kept denying that it meant something. So I stopped taking the Pill and got pregnant nearly straightaway. I thought, now he won't ever be able to forget me. He won't be able to pretend to our friends or his family that there wasn't really anything going on between us.'

On the positive side, in the case of many couples *both* partners want to have a child, as a physical bond between them, a living proof of their loving relationship. As one man put it, 'If we don't have a child there will be nothing to show that we were together or loved one another. If we have a child, somehow we will be joined forever.'

Couples often say they want a child because the child will be someone for them to love, who will also give them love in return. Some people want children to relive their happy childhood experiences, or sometimes to make up for the lack of them.

Sometimes people see children as important in forming a blood link between their families. 'Before, it was just "his family" and "my family". Now we have the children, we are all related to one another.'

MOTHERHOOD

There is no doubt that many women profoundly enjoy the experience of pregnancy, childbirth and motherhood. Some enjoy it so much that they have several children, in an age where having two is considered the norm and anything above this rather exceptional. Many women find being pregnant exciting and rewarding, despite physical discomforts such as morning sickness or the heaviness of late pregnancy. One mother said:

'I love my body when I'm pregnant. It seems round, full, complete somehow. I find that I am emotionally on an even keel throughout; no more pre-menstrual depressions and upsets. I love the sensation of a baby moving. I love the feeling that I am never alone, yet at the same time I am my own person. If I could always be five months pregnant, life would be bliss.'

Childbirth can be a woman's greatest experience despite the pain which is often emphasised to the exclusion of almost all else. Breastfeeding, too, can be a powerful physical experience and an emotional bond which provides immense rewards. Again, a mother talks of her feelings about these experiences: 'It's such a tremendous thing, you can't imagine what life will be like when it's all behind you. Nowadays we are conditioned to the idea that it's sexual intercourse which is all important, and that we mustn't be without it. Yet I've found pregnancy, childbirth and breastfeeding just as pleasurable as sex. When I weaned my last baby it was terrible; as if someone said, well that's it, you'll never have sex again.'

Of course, the satisfaction that children bring are not only felt on a physical or emotional level. In many developing countries people want children also because they are their wealth – especially sons – and will bring money into the family to help their parents in old age. Even though that does not really apply in most developed countries where there is state provision for the elderly, people are often still afraid of how they will fare in old age if they have no children. Needs are by no means only financial, either. In old age childless couples may feel alone and isolated, with no children or grandchildren to visit them or keep them in touch with the world. They may have good friends and neighbours, but it is not the same:

'There isn't anyone I feel I can ask to help me. If I ask the neighbours to do something for me, I feel that I have to do something back, like taking their cat in when they're late home and giving her supper, or giving them apples from the garden. It's only family you can ask things as of right, and now I have no family. If something happened to me, there would be no-one for them to ring, no-one to come to the bedside. Without family, who will care?'

People have always looked to their children for security in their old age, and though nowadays not all children are prepared to take on the problems of elderly parents, many do. At any rate, children are people to look after your affairs if you become less able to look after them yourself and people to turn to in a crisis, to leave your possessions to, to organise your funeral.

LOVED AND LOVING

People also want children because of a natural and powerful need to give and receive love. In our society we tend to have only a few truly intimate relationships, often restricted to the immediate family. If a couple have no children, they may have only one another to love, and can seem too great a burden to put on one another.

Children both need and give a great deal of physical affection, fulfilling the parents' need to touch and hold as well as their own. A happy household with children in it is full of noise, warmth, activity, hugs and kisses. Caring for their children gives parents a sense of warmth and security; making someone else feel safe makes us feel safe too. As one mother recalls, 'I never felt so happy as when they were small and I would tuck them into bed in the evening. I could make everything all right for them, and that made me feel that everything else in the world was right, too.'

Children also provide so much work and activity that there is little time for parents to wonder what the purpose of their lives is. The children need them; that is enough. Festivals like Christmas or birthdays take on a new meaning because they are done for the children. The children's response to them makes them magic, and we recall our own feelings in childhood before we became aware of the commercialisation of such holidays.

WANTING TOO MUCH

People who have had a happy childhood may want to relive the same pleasures with their children. People whose childhoods have not been happy may also want children so that they can create the happy childhood that they were denied. This may seem very important as a means to heal the wounds of the past. Yet sometimes these parents may focus so much on making their children happy that they see their children too much as a route to their own fulfilment. This can poison parent-child relationships and make things go badly wrong.

Parents who see children as extensions of themselves and try to make their children achieve the goals they wanted to achieve – but often failed or lacked the opportunity to pursue – seldom achieve the satisfaction they seek and may instead alienate their children. Children whose parents focus too much on what they achieve may feel that they are not loved for themselves, only for what they can do. The insecurity created may make the child reject his work or behave badly in order to test whether his parents will still love him nonetheless.

Some people who have had a child or children after years of infertility, or with the help of new fertility techniques, view their children as even more important to them, and find it harder to let go of them when they reach adolescence. There is some evidence that this is true of adopted children (see Chapter 4). There is a danger that in wanting so much to have a 'baby', one forgets the child and then the adult the baby becomes. In the words of one woman who had test-tube twins at the fourth attempt, 'The fertility treatment is so demanding that you lose all sight of what it's for. I found myself suddenly asking, what if I don't even like parenthood at the end of all this?'

Let this woman's comment lead us into the next chapter, which looks at the causes and treatment of infertility, and the emotions and experience of those who are infertile but most certainly do want children.

2

Infertility: causes, tests and treatments

Infertility is usually defined as the inability of a couple to conceive a child after a year of regular sexual intercourse. In fact, many couples who are 'infertile' by this definition will conceive eventually – either naturally or following infertility treatment. Infertility is a widespread problem – as many as one in six couples will consult their doctor because they are worried about not having conceived. Today, infertility may seem even harder to bear by a generation accustomed to using contraception, planning births – almost to the month – and having more choices and more control over their lives.

HOW CONCEPTION OCCURS

Human conception is a miraculous and complex event, and what is surprising is perhaps that pregnancy occurs so often, rather than that it sometimes fails. A human egg is released every month from a woman's ovary under the influence of a complex cycle of hormones released by the pituitary gland and the hypothalamus. The egg is swept into the fallopian tubes by the delicate projections (the fimbriae) at the end of the tubes, where it is normally fertilised by the man's sperm. The fertilised egg then moves down the tube and, aided by the tiny hair-like cilia which line the tube, enter the womb. The embryo

15

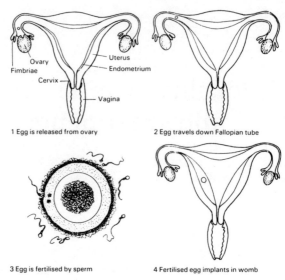

1 Egg is released from ovary

2 Egg travels down Fallopian tube

3 Egg is fertilised by sperm

4 Fertilised egg implants in womb

How conception occurs

must implant into the lining of the womb (the endometrium) where it starts to produce hormones which will stimulate its growth. The body in the ovary, the corpus luteum, from which the egg was released, must produce enough of the hormone progesterone to sustain the pregnancy until, after the first three months, the placenta takes over. The woman's womb must be structurally sound and capable of expanding to contain the growing foetus and the cervix strong enough to hold the baby in until it is ready to be born.

It is estimated that it takes a fertile couple having regular sexual intercourse an average of six months to conceive. At any stage, something can go wrong and a pregnancy will not result:

- Sometimes an egg will not be released;
- The egg and sperm may fail to meet and fertilise.
- Many early embryos fail to implant and sometimes an implanted embryo fails to develop or is rejected by the mother's body.
- An abnormality in the foetus or a lack of sufficient levels of the hormone progesterone may make it impossible for the embryo to survive, resulting in a miscarriage.

Roughly 30 per cent of infertility is caused by a problem in the woman; 30 per cent in the man; 30 per cent by both and about 10 per cent is unexplained. These figures are repeated in almost every guide to the subject, yet in reality, the figures may be somewhat different. A recent survey at the Bristol Maternity Hospital showed the main causes of infertility to be ovulatory failure (21 per cent), tubal damage (14 per cent), and sperm defects (24 per cent); 28 per cent had unexplained infertility. Unexplained infertility has tended to fall with better diagnosis and an improved understanding of what causes infertility, but is still more common than many doctors like to admit.

CAUSES OF INFERTILITY IN WOMEN

Any woman who fears that she is infertile and yet wants a child, should first see her doctor. The problem may be easily diagnosed and treatment begun without any delay. Some treatments are quite simple; for example, if the woman is not ovulating, a course of fertility drugs can be given to see if these will activate her ovaries. There are several fertility drugs, and while the doctor may know which is the best to try, often he simply has to go through each in turn, trying different doses, to see what is successful or not. This can have the effect of making the woman feel like a human guinea pig.

VISITING A FERTILITY CLINIC

If they eventually visit a fertility clinic, both partners will be asked for details of their medical history: any past illnesses and any surgery. They will also be asked questions about their sex life; how many sexual partners they have had, how often they make love, and so on. Many people find this an intrusion into their privacy, but it is all very relevant.

A routine physical examination will then be carried out on

both partners. They will be examined to check that their respective reproductive organs are normal. For the man, this means inspecting the external genitals and in particular the testicles for any signs of a varicocele or other abnormality. The woman will have an internal pelvic examination, during which the doctor will insert a speculum to hold the walls of the vagina apart so that he can view the cervix and take swabs for testing if he suspects a vaginal infection. He will also use his hands to feel the internal organs; this may enable him to detect problems such as fibroids, ovarian cysts or scarring from previous infections.

Tests undergone by the woman

One of the first tests for infertility is to find out whether the woman is ovulating, using basal body temperature charts. At the time of ovulation there is a small but distinct rise in the body's temperature, due to production of the hormone progesterone. This can be measured by taking a woman's temperature every morning on waking up, a procedure which many find irksome. A three-monthly record should show if you are ovulating and if your cycle is normal, though you may be asked to continue keeping a temperature chart for much longer than this. Because temperature charts are sometimes difficult to interpret and are not always reliable, the woman will probably be given further tests to measure the level of hormones which control ovulation. A blood progesterone test, which is a simple and painless way of measuring the level of progesterone when it reaches its peak at about day 24 in a 28 day cycle, can be done. If the level of progesterone is high, it is a good indication that ovulation has occurred.

THE POST-COITAL TEST may also pinpoint why a woman is not conceiving. The woman makes an appointment for the time of the month when she thinks she will be ovulating. The couple are asked to have sexual intercourse on the night before or the morning of the appointment. At the clinic, the doctor will take a sample of the woman's cervical mucus from the neck of the womb, for examination. The quality of the mucus – clear and slippery, or sticky and opaque – will tend to indicate whether the woman has ovulated. By examining the mucus under a microscope, it is also possible to tell if the sperm are normal, if there are enough of them and whether there are any antibodies against them. If post-coital tests are repeatedly not very good, the next step may be to test the semen and mucus for antibodies to sperm which may interfere with sperm motility.

ENDOMETRIAL BIOPSY This other procedure for assessing the woman's hormone levels involves taking a small sample of the lining of the womb for examination. This is a minor surgical procedure, similar to a D and C. The test should show if the womb lining is sufficiently primed by hormones to be able to receive the egg for implantation. If the woman is ovulating normally, the next line of investigation will be to see if the Fallopian tubes are clear.

A HYSTEROSALPINGRAM is an X-ray of the uterus and Fallopian tubes, for which purpose a dye is injected through the cervix and into the uterus. The dye passes through the womb, along the Fallopian tubes and into the pelvic cavity, enabling all the organs to be viewed. Some women may have a simpler test in which carbon dioxide gas is blown through the tubes to check if they are open; if so, the gas will enter the abdominal cavity, causing a pain under the shoulder blades, which fortunately soon wears off.

A LAPAROSCOPY is used to detect blocked or damaged tubes and other abnormalities of the womb or ovaries. Under general anaesthetic, a small incision is made in the navel and a laparoscope – a telescope-like instrument – is inserted which allows the surgeon to examine the organs in detail and assess the extent of any damage.

Tests undergone by the man

The man will be asked to produce one or more sperm samples, and this should be done at the outset, before the woman undergoes any major procedures. The man is asked to produce a sample by masturbation into a sterile container either in the clinic, or at home. If he does this at home, he must deliver the sample to the clinic within one-and-a-half hours. The sample is examined to see if the sperm are healthy, numerous and motile. Since one test is not always reliable, a poor result may mean he has to repeat the test. Sometimes a man is diagnosed as subfertile on the basis of one test alone. Yet a single sperm count is very unreliable as an indicator of a man's normal fertility. Sperm counts vary enormously from one act of intercourse to another. If all is well, this may be the only test the man has to undergo. If he has a very low or absent sperm count, however, investigations may be undertaken to see if a cause can be found. The sperm may also be examined by the post-coital test, which may give some insight into why the sperm are not functioning properly.

SCROTOTOMY
In some cases the man may have a scrototomy, an operation carried out under general anaesthetic to open up the scrotum and see whether there are any abnormalities or obstructions.

Aftermath of contraception

Contraceptive methods are a cause of infertility only very rarely. The inter-uterine device (IUD) can increase a woman's chance of suffering from pelvic inflammatory disease, which can lead to infertility. The contraceptive Pill sometimes leads to a condition called post-Pill amenorrhoea, in which a woman's periods do not return when she stops the Pill – research has shown that this only lasts for a maximum of two years after Pill use, and it can also be treated with drugs.

A woman used to taking the Pill for several years, or using an IUD or cap regularly and worrying every time her period is late, may well expect to get pregnant as soon as she stops using her chosen contraception – but often does not. This does not necessarily mean that she is infertile. However, as a woman gets older her fertility declines, and using contraception for years may mean she is less fertile when she stops and tries to get pregnant. Also, using contraception, and particularly the Pill, can disguise infertility problems for years; the Pill usually means that a woman has a regular cycle and so may not realise she is not capable of ovulating.

Hormonal problems

One of the most common causes of infertility in women is a malfunctioning of the complex hormonal interactions which govern a woman's menstrual cycle. The woman's monthly cycle is controlled by the pituitary gland in the brain which, in turn, is governed by another gland called the hypothalamus. The pituitary produces a follicle-stimulating hormone (FSH), which controls the production of the hormone oestrogen by the ovary. It also prepares one of the follicles inside the ovary to release the egg. A second pituitary hormone, luteinising hormone (LH), enables the ovary to release its egg. Oestrogen causes the lining of the womb to thicken in readiness to receive the fertilised egg.

If the egg is not fertilised, the corpus luteum begins to shrink, levels of oestrogen and progesterone decrease, the lining of the womb disintegrates and menstrual bleeding results. The falling levels of oestrogen and progesterone stimulate the pituitary to produce more FSH, and the cycle begins again.

If the egg is fertilised, however, and implants into the womb, the corpus luteum continues to produce oestrogen and progesterone until the placenta attaching the foetus to the wall of the womb is mature enough to produce the necessary hormones itself.

Failure to ovulate is normally caused by the woman's body failing to produce enough of the pituitary hormones, or releasing them at the wrong time. Since the pituitary is ultimately controlled by the hypothalamus, anything which affects the hypothalamus can also affect this gland. The hypothalamus can be affected by severe physical and emotional stress, as many women will know when the stress of travel, work, illness or emotional turmoil disrupts their menstrual cycle.

TREATMENT
Help for women unable to ovulate has been available for

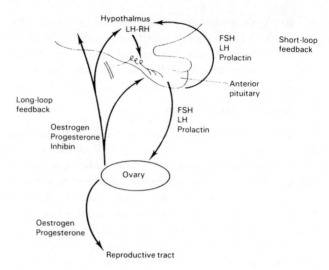

The hormonal interactions which govern the menstrual cycle.

many years in the form of fertility drugs. There are two main types: those which prod the pituitary into producing FSH and LH on time and those which replace FSH and LH if this approach fails:

• **Clomiphene (Clomid)** is an artificial drug which triggers the release of FSH and LH in the pituitary. It seems to induce ovulation in about 80 per cent of women treated, though not all these will succeed in getting pregnant. One reason for this is that clomiphene tends to prevent the cervical mucus from becoming fluid at the fertile time in the month to enable the sperm to enter the womb. This problem can sometimes be overcome by giving oestrogen as well in the few days before ovulation.

Sometimes a combination of clomiphene and human chorionic gonadotrophin (HCG, a hormone produced by the young embryo) given on the fourteenth day of the cycle will induce women to ovulate who would not do so on clomiphene alone.

Clomiphene also seems to help women with a progesterone deficiency.

Clomiphene (Clomid) has been in use for many years and is considered safe, although a few women do have unpleasant side-effects, such as nausea, feeling bloated, or very rarely, enlargement of the ovaries accompanied by pain in the pelvis. Some infertility specialists deny the severity of these symptoms, or fail to inform women of them.

Recently there has been some concern that clomiphene might cause an increase in the number of eggs released following its use which have chromosomal abnormalities. Others have questioned whether there might be other long-term effects on the children who are conceived after their mothers took fertility drugs, as happened with women who took the drug DES (diethylstilboestrel) in early pregnancy to prevent a miscarriage. This is of particular concern to women who take large doses of fertility drugs to make them produce more than one egg, or superovulate, as is done for IVF and other treatments. However, there is no evidence to support such fears as yet.

- **Human menopausal gonadotrophin, (HMG), or Pergonal**, is a hormone extracted from the urine of pregnant women and prepares the follicles which release the egg to ripen. It is usually given with an injection of another drug, HCG, which actually triggers ovulation. About 90 per cent of women will ovulate with this treatment, though again not all will conceive and some will miscarry. About 20 to 30 per cent of pregnancies resulting from this treatment will be twins or more; HMG is responsible for most of the multiple pregnancies which occur with fertility drugs.

The hormone HMG is very potent and may also overstimulate the ovaries, so its level in the blood and urine needs to be monitored daily. A new development which might overcome this problem is a small 'pump' about the size of a pocket book which, attached to the woman's arm, provides small, even doses of hormone through a fine needle. However, having a pump attached day and night and having to go and have the needle repositioned when necessary can be unpleasant.

For women who do not ovulate with either of these drugs, there may be hope with a drug called bromo-criptine. Some women do not ovulate because they have in their blood a high level of a hormone called prolactin, which is normally only produced in quantity while women are breastfeeding and tends to prevent ovulation. Bromocriptine prevents the pituitary from producing prolactin, and after treatment with it ovulation occurs in about 95 per cent of women who previously produced too much prolactin.

Scarring or structural abnormalities

The other major causes of infertility in women are scarring of the reproductive organs by past disease or surgery, or struc-tural abnormalities present from birth.

- Untreated sexually transmitted diseases, especially gonor-rhoea, can result in infertility. As many as 80 per cent of infected women never have any severe symptoms with the disease, and may not realise that they have it and infection has spread to the Fallopian tubes, causing damage.
- PID (pelvic inflammatory disease) which can start after an induced abortion or miscarriage, after childbirth, after surgery in the pelvic region or after infection with a sexually transmitted disease, can cause tubal scarring and blockage.
- Other infections which can affect fertility are chlamydia and mycoplasmas. Chlamydia, a bacterium which closely resem-bles a large virus, has deceptively mild symptoms and an untreated 'silent' infection can destroy the inside of a woman's Fallopian tubes in a matter of days. Mycoplasmas, another organism, may affect fertility and has been held responsible for miscarriages.

Other Causes

Endometriosis is a disease which may affect as many as five to ten per cent of women at some stage in their reproductive lives. The condition is caused by patches of the endometrial tissue which lines the womb, or endometrium, becoming deposited outside the womb. This tissue, like the womb lining, thickens and bleeds with each menstrual cycle. Scar tissue is then formed which may block the ends of the Fallopian tubes, or adhesions may form which prevent the tube from picking up the egg on its release from the ovary.

Endometriosis can be treated by a number of drugs; birth control pills or progesterone, or a drug called Danazol, which blocks production of the two pituitary hormones. The idea is that these treatments 'switch off' the menstrual cycle, stopping the patches of endometrial tissue from bleeding; they will then fade away, and any adhesions or scar tissue can be removed by careful surgery.

FIBROIDS OR POLYPS IN THE WOMB are benign growths which can affect fertility by growing to a size large enough to cause blockage or prevent the egg implanting and growing. These can be removed by surgery.

MALFORMATIONS OF THE WOMB, such as the presence of a dividing wall or septum, again can sometimes be corrected by surgery.

• A further cause of damage to the tubes is previous surgery in the abdominal region. Bleeding or trauma to the tissues may result in the formation of scar tissue or adhesions which may then block or fix the tubes, ovaries or womb into unnatural positions that make it impossible for the egg to pass from the ovaries into the Fallopian tubes, making conception impossible. One leading British microsurgeon who has specialised in repairing damaged Fallopian tubes has criticized surgeons for not taking enough care when operating in the abdominal region of women of childbearing age. Of 108 women with tubal damage referred to the Hammersmith Hospital, London over a three-month period, 73 per cent had had previous pelvic surgery.

Increasing skill in carrying out delicate microsurgery has given more women with blocked Fallopian tubes a chance to achieve pregnancy. However, if surgery is not effective, there is still hope through the test-tube baby treatment or IVF (see Chapter 4).

TUBAL OR ECTOPIC PREGNANCY

Occasionally a fertilised egg fails to move down through the tube and into the womb and, instead, grows in the tube. Eventually it will burst the tube, causing considerable bleeding and damage.

An ectopic pregnancy thus results in both the loss of one pregnancy and a possible barrier to future conception. One tube is almost inevitably lost and the other may be damaged by bleeding caused by the tube rupturing or surgery to remove the pregnancy. It is estimated that about fifty per cent of women who have an ectopic pregnancy may never conceive again.

Often an ectopic pregnancy occurs when there has been some damage to the tube, perhaps caused by past infections or surgery. It is also more common if a woman becomes pregnant with an IUD in place. An ectopic pregnancy is very painful and can be life-threatening. However, prompt medical attention to remove the developing egg before the tube can burst avoids many risks as well as improving the chances of successfully reconstructing the damaged tube.

Multiple early miscarriage

This is another problem which is now being recognised as a cause of infertility. Some women are able to produce eggs that are fertilised and even begin to implant into the lining of the womb, but then fail to develop further, resulting in an early miscarriage. At one time most women to whom this happened probably did not ever realise that they had conceived. With early, sensitive pregnancy tests that allow a woman to know she has conceived even before her period is late, many more women are realising that they have suffered an early pregnancy loss.

Miscarriages are very common – about one in seven pregnancies are estimated to end in miscarriage, and the figure would probably be even higher if all early pregnancy losses were detected and included. About half of them are caused by abnormalities in the foetus that prevent further growth. Miscarriages are more common in first pregnancies and some doctors think that these pregnancies are a kind of 'trial run'. The risk of miscarriage increases with age, and miscarriages following fertility treatment are also more common than in other women.

Most women who suffer one or even two miscarriages go on to have a normal pregnancy. Only after three successive miscarriages do the risks of having another go up substantially. Some women however have repeated miscarriages, and seem unable to carry a baby to term. Sometimes this happens because the woman or her partner are carrying a chromosomal abnormality. It has recently been recognised, however, that some women miscarry because they are rejecting the baby in their womb as foreign. In a normal pregnancy, the woman's immune system is activated in such a way that she does not recognise the baby as a foreign body and reject it. Some women and their partners seem to be a poor genetic match, so that partner's baby will always be rejected. Immunising the woman with an injection of her partner's white blood cells can overcome this rejection problem and allow her to have a normal pregnancy and baby.

INFERTILITY IN MEN

Male infertility can also be caused by blocked tubes, the vasa deferentia, which carry sperm from the testes where they are made to the penis. Tubes can be blocked for any of the following reasons:

- From birth due to a congenital defect.
- Through scarring caused by sexually transmitted diseases.
- Through surgery, as in a vasectomy.

Male infertility can also be caused by:

- Undescended testicles – if these are not diagnosed early in a boy's life permanent infertility will result.
- By infections involving the testicles; orchitis, inflammation of the testicles following mumps, very occasionally can result in infertility.
- Varicocele – a sort of varicose vein of the testicle – is a common cause of male infertility.

- Rarely, disorders of ejaculation are responsible for male infertility. Sometimes, as a result of illness such as diabetes or surgery such as a prostatectomy, sperm is ejaculated backwards into the bladder at orgasm.
- Male infertility is also the result of a low sperm count, or of a large proportion of the man's sperm being abnormal. Although research is being done, no-one really understands the causes of low sperm counts; however, their origin is believed to be hormonal.

TREATMENTS

Because so little is understood about the causes of much male infertility, very limited help is available for the majority of men with a low or absent sperm count. Some causes are known (see above) but there is little to be done about them.

The most curable form of male infertility is that caused by a varicocele, or varicose vein, around the testicle. A simple operation to tie off the vein results in an improvement to sperm quantity and quality in about two-thirds of cases, thus increasing the chances of conception.

Blocked or scarred vasa deferentia, especially after vasectomy, may be restored surgically but there is only a 50 per cent success rate; this is because a man with blocked tubes often produces antibodies to the sperm as they cannot be ejaculated and have to be reabsorbed by the body.

Other causes of a low sperm count are very resistant to treatment. Various hormone treatments have been tried, but with a very low success rate. Some studies have shown that the success rate is actually lower among treated men than among those who have not received any drugs at all. Many of the drugs – some of which are the same as female fertility drugs – also have unpleasant side-effects such as loss of libido, swollen breasts or loss of body hair. To a man whose self-esteem is already dented by the fact of his infertility, these side-effects can be impossible to bear.

One new technique that may help men with a low sperm count, is the split ejaculate technique, where the first part of several ejaculates – the part richest in sperm – is pooled and introduced into the vagina through artificial insemination. This may not work, however, where a large number of abnormal sperm are present.

Now IVF and similar techniques such as GIFT offer new hope for subfertile men (see Chapter 4 for full details). Far fewer sperm are needed to achieve fertilisation in vitro, as the sperm do not have to make their arduous journey through the vagina, cervix, womb and tubes, with most being left behind at one stage or another.

Sometimes sperm are capable of fertilising an egg but not of penetrating the cervix or surviving long in the woman's reproductive tract. By mixing sperm directly with the egg, as in IVF, these problems may be overcome.

SELF-HELP
Some men can improve sperm counts with a healthier diet, stopping or reducing smoking and drinking alcohol, avoiding hot baths and not wearing tight underwear.

Since the testes are very sensitive to heat, men who work in a very hot environment sometimes experience a reduction in fertility; this can also sometimes be avoided.

Sperm counts can also be lowered by illness, especially involving a fever; sperm counts can be reduced for some time afterwards since it takes three months for sperm to be produced in the body. Fortunately, this is a short-term problem that will resolve itself.

OTHER POSSIBLE TREATMENTS
If the measures described in this chapter fail, or if the sperm count is consistently so low that conception is very unlikely, the main alternative is artificial insemination by donor (AID) (see Chapter 4).

Going through the tests and treatments already described is in itself a remarkable testament to most couple's desire for a child they can call their own. By the time these couples come to consider assisted reproduction techniques, they have probably already been through months or years of tests and the more orthodox fertility treatments. At the same time, it can be difficult to call a halt.

'You feel you've already invested so many years and so much pain in all this, you just have to go on to the end,' said one woman.

3

Facing up to infertility

Infertility is a difficult problem because many people feel that they are personally responsible for it. Having had an abortion in the past, delaying having a baby till later in life, using a method of contraception which may have affected fertility, can all haunt the infertile.

If infertility is unexplained – as about 10 per cent of it is – the couple may wonder if there is a psychological element. Couples are told to 'Relax, then you will conceive.' Some doctors and psychiatrists do believe that stress and anxiety can block conception.

One biochemist, Paul Entwhistle at Liverpool University, claims that 65 per cent of around 200 patients who had tried conventional infertility treatments conceived after hypnotherapy. He believes that a woman may 'switch off' her fertility subconsciously, failing to ovulate or making her tubes go into spasm, or affecting the blood supply in her womb, and so preventing implantation. This may explain why some women conceive after a dramatic event like moving home, starting a new job, or adopting a child, and why the chances of getting pregnant after a single act of rape seem higher than after a single act of sex in a consenting relationship – the shock may prevent the woman 'switching off' her fertility.

Obviously the mind and body are closely linked, and depression and anxiety clearly do have effects on fertility. A loss of interest in sex causes drying up of the vaginal secretions

31

that help sperm motility; it also reduces rates of sexual intercourse.

However, most psychological explanations of infertility concentrate on the woman; I have never seen a single suggestion that anxiety, stress or deep-seated fear of fatherhood might cause a man to have a low sperm count. The fact that people, especially women, often blame themselves for their infertility may make the stress of infertility far worse for them. Being considered to be neurotic or psychologically unstable – and even partially responsible for their condition – does not help a couple who want to have a child and seek treatment to realise that aim.

Infertility can also isolate people: from friends or contemporaries with children, and even from their families who may not understand. One infertile woman remembers the pain of hearing her mother say that she would have to advertise for some grandchildren; she was clearly hurt by her daughter's infertility but could not share the pain with her. Others find that friends and neighbours assume that they have chosen to be childless. Some are told they are 'lucky' to be childless or that they should 'make the best of it'. Infertility is little understood and is considered embarrassing to many because it implies sexual inadequacy of some kind. It often turns people in on themselves because they feel they cannot share their pain with others.

SOME REACTIONS TO INFERTILITY

Whatever the cause of infertility, the dawning realisation that having a baby may be difficult or impossible is very traumatic for most people. Infertility is one of the worst experiences many people have to cope with in their whole lives. Those who discover that they are infertile speak of it as a terrible blow, as bad for some as receiving the news that they are to lose part of their body or have a potentially terminal illness. One woman shows this clearly, when she recalls the feelings she had on receiving her diagnosis: 'They told me not only that I couldn't have children but that I had cancer. The first thing that struck me was grief that I couldn't have a baby. The fact that I also had cancer hit me about 30 seconds later.'

In Robert and Elizabeth Snowden's book, *The Gift of a Child*, a husband described his reactions on being told he was infertile. 'Anyone who's never actually been told, you can't tell them the feeling that you get. It's like being hit with a sledge-hammer . . . I never felt so ill in my life. It took me a long while to get over it.'

With men in particular, the discovery of infertility can trigger problems with sexuality. One American doctor who studied the reactions of men recently informed of their infertility found that almost two-thirds suffered a period of impotence lasting one to three months after hearing this news.

Anger, resentment and guilt

Jenny Hunt, an infertility counsellor at the Hammersmith Hospital, London, says that many couples have what might seem quite extreme reactions to the discovery of infertility. Many experience a loss of self-image, and may even hate themselves. They may hate their bodies, and in particular their genitals, which they feel are useless and have betrayed them.

One woman said that she hated her body, it seemed so ugly and useless. 'I remember saying to the consultant, well that's it then, I might as well have a double mastectomy and a hyster-ectomy now. What use is my womb and what use are my breasts if I will never use them to carry or feed a baby? He didn't understand me at all. He just seemed very shocked at my response.'

Such reactions may sound excessive, but they are not unusual. Many infertile people have self-mutilating fantasies, due to the anger they feel towards their bodies for letting them down.

Sometimes one partner feels anger at the other one for being infertile. Jenny Hunt says that most wives of infertile husbands feel angry with them and hate themselves for it. Others, male and female, feel that if they are the one responsible for the infertility problem, their partner should feel free to divorce them and find someone else. 'If I can't have (or give you) children, feel free to go and find someone who can,' is the common cry.

Depression and grief

Many infertile couples need help in working through their very understandable emotions. Many of the problems can be overcome when a couple have genuinely accepted their infertility, or have found ways around it. But at the time, this may seem impossible. Depression may set in and occasionally an infertile woman turns her depression inwards and attempts suicide. For such women, having a baby has become more important even than life itself.

The grief felt by infertile couples is of a very particular kind. Unlike the loss of a parent, relative, child or loved one, when a couple are infertile they grieve the loss of a person they have never known. Normally when a person grieves they have memories to treasure and to comfort them, but an infertile couple have only lost hopes and fantasies. Even so, they go through all the usual phases of grief – denial, anger, mourning, acceptance. Because with many forms of infertility there is always a small hope that the couple will succeed, some people get stuck somewhere in the grieving process. Others have their hopes awoken again, and this makes it much more difficult to accept a final 'negative' diagnosis.

As one mother said, 'People were always trotting out to me stories of women who had finally conceived after years and years of waiting. "Oh, so-and-so, down the road, she had to wait six years and then she had this beautiful baby boy." Or, "What about this test-tube baby thing, have you tried that?" They are always trying to give you hope when you know you should give up. I used to cling to every story I heard about people having babies against innumerable odds, as I so much wanted to believe that there was hope. It made adjusting to the whole problem so much harder.'

STRESSES OF TREATMENT

Although the fact of infertility itself is hard to bear, it is made worse by the way in which infertility services are usually provided and by the tests and treatments which are offered. The stress involved can weigh a couple down, and hoping can in itself be a terrible strain.

As one mother of one, desperate to have a second baby, explained: 'You need an incredible commitment to get through it all. At one stage, when I was having blood tests and cervical mucus tests and everything, I had to be at the hospital at eight-thirty every morning for weeks on end. That needs great commitment when you are really busy. Trailing backwards and forwards and making arrangements for the child – and for my husband Tom to be late at work. Other people had to be there at eight-thirty in the morning, too. It certainly weeded out the people who really wanted a baby. I don't regret the time and emotional energy we put into it now, because in the end we did have Jack. But I think that if we hadn't I would regret it terribly.'

Because of the shortage of infertility clinics (see Chapter 5) many people have to travel long distances to receive help. Many hospitals do not have a special clinic, so infertile patients have to queue with other women, sometimes pregnant, sometimes seeking abortions. This can add to the pain of their own situation, as can the waiting. Because the infertility specialists have so many patients, they often cannot give enough time to each couple to explore their anxieties and fears or explain the tests and treatments fully to them. So infertile couples often little understand what is going on or what the treatment they are getting is supposed to do. Frequently in researching this book I was given information about a couple's treatment which I knew could not possibly be correct.

During interviews with a specialist, many couples found it hard to take in what was being said. 'I knew we would get the result of the sperm test – I could see it sitting on his desk. But instead of telling us straightaway, he went on talking for ten to fifteen minutes. I couldn't take in a word. I kept trying to peer at this piece of paper and see what it said. When I finally asked him, he said, "Oh yes, that was fine." But it would have helped if he'd told us that to begin with.

'He said that I didn't seem to be ovulating and went on to suggest tests and treatments. But he didn't pause after this devastating bit of information, to give me a chance to react. So instead of listening to what he was saying, I just sat there trying to keep back the tears. After all, this was the first time I'd been given any confirmation that there really was something wrong with me.'

Effect on sexuality

Almost all infertile couples speak of the problems they have in their sexual lives. Sexuality is no longer an expression of joy and pleasure in one another, it is a source of grief. One woman says, 'It seemed so pointless to go on having sex when you knew that nothing was ever going to come of it.'

Many couples' sex lives are ruined at least for a time by their desperate attempts to conceive. They are not helped in this by much of the medical advice that couples are given on improving the chances of conception occurring. The sort of advice infertile couples receive is as follows:

- Intercourse should be timed to the most fertile time in a woman's monthly cycle, i.e. the two or three days before the egg is released by the ovary.
- The woman should stay lying on her back for up to half an hour after intercourse, to give the sperm the maximum chance of getting into the womb.
- Certain positions for intercourse are helpful.
- Sometimes couples are told to try artificial insemination at home with the man's sperm, which they will be taught how to do at the clinic. There is little evidence that in the vast majority of cases this will be any improvement on natural conception.

All of this advice and its conscientious practise may cause havoc to a couple's sex life and actually further reduce their chance of starting a pregnancy, as sex becomes a task to be performed rather than a pleasure. It often becomes less and less frequent, too.

The infertility tests themselves can be very time-consuming and intrusive. Because many have to be carried out at a certain time in the month, normally at around ovulation, they have to be spaced out over many months. Sometimes the tests interfere with the chance of normal conception, so some specialists specify longer gaps in between to allow the couple chance to conceive naturally.

Some tests demand making love to order. For example, for the postcoital test the couple are asked to make love on waking in the morning and, afterwards, for the woman to come straight to the clinic so that her cervical mucus can be examined to see how the sperm are surviving in it. To be at the clinic within a specified time after making love can be difficult if you do not live close to the clinic. Also, by no means everyone can 'perform' to order like this, and if they fail another precious month is wasted.

Men's reactions

The pressure of these tests is often worse for the man. He is expected to produce several sperm samples for the clinic, and told to make love to his wife at a certain time. Some men find the pressure to 'perform' in such circumstances intolerable. 'I started to find I just couldn't get turned on or get an erection on nights when it was "expected" of me. I just couldn't feel anything but, oh no not this again. So I took to staying late at work on the nights when we were supposed to try to conceive. Sarah didn't understand, she just got mad at me and said that I was letting her down. She had to go through all these tests and I couldn't even make love to her when it was expected.'

For some infertility treatments, such as in vitro fertilisation (IVF), the man is expected to produce a sperm sample in order to coincide with the operation to retrieve his wife's eggs from her ovary. Men at the Hammersmith Hospital, London, whose wives are undergoing IVF have to queue in a corridor outside the male lavatory to take turns in producing the sample. It is not surprising under these conditions that some men cannot produce a sperm sample or even get an erection at all.

Some clinics now have in reserve a frozen sample of the man's sperm, to take some of the pressure off him, and so that there is some of his own sperm available if he does fail, although IVF fertilisation is less successful with frozen sperm. There have been cases where, instead, the couple have been offered donor sperm and, under the stress involved, have been rushed into saying 'yes' to avoid postponing the IVF procedure and possibly wasting the collected eggs. They might later regret this decision if it was after all possible for them to have had their own child.

Women's reactions

Some of the tests for the woman involve surgical procedures (see Chapters 2 and 4) which can be painful or unpleasant. In one test carbon dioxide gas is passed through the tubes to see if it passes freely – if so the woman feels a pain in her shoulder caused by gas in the abdominal cavity, though the gas is quickly absorbed by the body. 'They told me this test might be painful but not how painful,' says one woman.

Another test is a hysterosalpingram, an X-ray of the womb and tubes. A small quantity of dye is injected into the womb and tubes, then an X-ray is taken to show if there are any blockages or distortions of the womb or tubes. If there is no blockage, the dye will pass into the tubes and then into the abdominal cavity where it is absorbed. Most women experience cramping rather like a bad period pain with this test, although the extent varies; some women find it tolerable, others extremely painful. Sometimes one or both tubes go into spasm during this test, giving the impression that they are blocked when they are not. Sometimes, giving a muscle relaxant overcomes this problem.

A typical story

Many couples' attempts to have a child last over many years of infertility tests and treatment, attempts to adopt or find alternatives. The desperate lengths to which some couples are prepared to go shows how deep is the need to have a child. Mike and Gena Dodd faced years of infertility before they finally found a solution to their childlessness with a surrogate mother. Their story is typical of many.

'I had my appendix out when I was 19; it didn't seem very important at the time. I never thought about it when we decided to start a family. In 1970, after over a year of trying to start a family, we went to our GP. Eventually we got an appointment at the hospital. Tests showed that Mike's sperm count was low but that he was still fertile. I had various tests. the doctor told me he would insert dye into my Fallopian tubes to see if they were open. It was very painful, and I could not concentrate on what the doctor said ... later I learned that my tubes were clear.

'It was decided to try the fertility drug, half strength Clomid. Then we moved to Scotland and I went for an appointment at the new hospital ... the doctor examined me and told me I would never get pregnant. I was dumb-founded. He did not give me any explanation and I was shown the door.

'We decided to try to adopt and were placed on the Adoption Resource Exchange list for hard-to-place children in 1975. Then in 1976 we tried artificial insemination with husband's sperm (AIH). After the insemination I had violent pains ... I went into hospital and they found a cyst on my left ovary, so they had to remove part of the ovary. I found out then that I had had my right ovary removed with my appendix when I was 19. I was told this was routine procedure if they found something wrong with it ... no-one had thought to inform me of it at the time.

'I then considered the test-tube baby treatment, IVF, but couldn't have it because Steptoe said he was only doing it with people who had two perfectly good ovaries. In the meantime we went on with temperature charts and trying to conceive, but thought adoption was our best hope.

'So, in 1977 we wrote to more adoption agencies. A year later we had an assessment – after another six months we were finally interviewed for the first time by the senior social worker. In 1978, I again had violent pain and another cyst on the ovary was discovered – this one burst and I had an emergency operation. While I was in hospital Mike 'phoned to say we had been accepted by the adoption agency. I cried with joy, I might only have half an ovary but we were back on the list for a baby.

'We were told that two babies were coming up for adoption. We waited on tenterhooks for three months but no word came. I phoned up but the social worker seemed to have forgotten what she had told me. She just said that at present there were no babies for adoption and none coming up in the near future.

'Mike sought help with a drink problem (neither of us considered it serious, he just thought he should get help before it did become so). The agency wrote and said they wanted our medical reports updated, so of course it came up. We were taken off the adoption agency list.

'We started to challenge this decision, writing to the social work department, the agency, our MP. Then my hopes were raised ... my period was two days late. The following day I had pains again and once more went into hospital. The doctor said he thought it was best if they removed the ovary completely, and they would have to remove my womb as well, but as I was only 34 they would prevent the change of life with drugs. I knew it was for the best but it was so final. No more hoping maybe one day, no more taking my temperature, nothing. For the next two hours before I went down to surgery I was left to my own thoughts, the anguish of knowing I would never have Mike's child, almost certainly never hold a baby in my arms, either Mike's or adopted.'

Gena and Mike Dodd finally succeeded in their 14-year quest for a baby when they had a baby boy through a surrogate mother in August 1984. More of this will be told in the next chapter.

Such persistence is not unusual. Many couples spend their lives one way or another trying to have a baby until they either succeed – naturally, through treatment or through adoption – in having a baby or finally accept that they are too old and that there is no more hope. Without children, life can seem empty. Couples may feel that they have no-one to whom they can give all the love they are capable of giving. One infertile woman says, 'I feel so frustrated – I could scream – because I know I would be a good mother, I have so much love inside me with nowhere to go.'

A KIND OF ACCEPTANCE

But for many couples, in the end, there is some kind of acceptance. Although they may always regret their infertility, they may find positive ways of coming to terms with it and finding fulfilment, or in involving themselves with children in other ways – through friends, godchildren, work or volunteering. Some people even find that the experience of coming to terms with infertility makes them feel wiser, more helpful and compassionate people. Indeed, for many, once the uncertainty of treatment is over, the worst pain is over too.

Catherine, who finally gave up treatment at the age of 42 after she was told her hopes were minimal, felt a great sense of liberation. 'If you had asked me about it three years ago, I would have been desperate. I had been trying for so long to have a baby that I couldn't accept the thought of failure. The worst is, our infertility had never fully been explained; there was always hope. Yet suddenly, when I admitted to myself that it just wasn't going to happen, I realised that in one way I didn't even want it to. I was becoming obsessed with my age, with being such an old parent, with the risks of having a handicapped baby, with the changes we would need to make to our lives. I actually feel freer and happier than I have done for years.'

Whether infertile people should try to come to terms with their infertility and find other sources of satisfaction in life or press on with medical treatment or explore other ways to have a child can be their decision alone. Those who succeed in having a baby will find the pain of infertility fades in the delight of a longed-for birth and family life. Those who fail will finally have to come to some kind of acceptance of their infertility and may regret the wasted years.

As one woman said, 'If I had known in the beginning that it wouldn't work for me, I would have said 'no' to all those tests, drugs and attempts at IVF. But I didn't know, so I spent years wrapped up in trying to have a baby; now I feel so much older and wearier that it's harder to think of something else

I could do – all those opportunities for jobs and training I turned down because infertility and IVF was ruling my whole life.'

Even if the attempt to have a child is successful, it is not without its regrets; 'I was biding time during that whole period of my life, not really enjoying anything, not really thinking about anything else . . . I still regret the waste of time involved – eight years out of my life – even though we did have a baby in the end.'

The advanced treatments such couples undertake are the subject of the next chapter.

4

New ways to parenthood

A decade has passed since the first 'test-tube baby', Louise Brown, entered the world on 25 July 1978. During that time the technique of in vitro fertilisation (IVF) has become established and new techniques have been developed from it; IVF is now just one of the many new ways in which the infertile can be helped to have their own child. The chart overleaf summarizes these new methods.

The new infertility treatments have become ever more important since the early 1970s because the great majority of couples unable to have a child have no hopes of adopting one either. The number of babies and children available for adoption has fallen dramatically due to the success of modern methods of contraception and the passing of such legislation as the British 1967 Abortion Act, which made abortions safe and legal. Also, more unmarried women have chosen to keep their babies as single motherhood has become more socially acceptable.

In the 1960s, nearly 20,000 children were adopted by strangers; by the early 1980s, the number of healthy white babies had fallen to less than 1,000.

This fall in the number of babies available has dramatically changed the prospects of couples wishing to adopt a baby. Because demand now far exceeds supply, waiting lists for healthy babies are long and arbitrary reasons are found to exclude groups of people – for example, those over 30 or under 20, and the previously divorced. Couples are given

43

THE NEW INFERTILITY TREATMENTS

SPERM	EGG	WOMB	MEANS OF CONCEPTION	TREATMENT
H	W	W	Natural	
H	W	W	AI	AIH
H	W	W	IVF	IVF
D	W	W	AI	AID
D	W	W	IVF	IVF with donor sperm
H	D	W	IVF	IVF with donor egg
D	D	W	IVF	IVF with donor embryo
H	S	S	AI/Natural	Surrogate motherhood
H	W	HM	IVF or AI + ET	Host mother
D	W	HM	IVF or AI + ET	Host mother with donor sperm
H	W	W	AI (posthumous)	AID (husband dead)
H	W	HM	IVF or AI + ET (posthumous)	Host mother (wife dead)
H	S	S	AI (posthumous)	Surrogate mother (husband dead)
H	D	HM	IVF or AI + ET	Host mother with donor egg
D	D	HM	IVF or AI + ET	Host mother with donor embryo
D	W	HM	IVF or AI + ET	Host mother wth donor sperm

KEY

H:	Husband (or partner)	HM:	Host mother
W:	Wife (or partner)	AI:	Artificial Insemination
D:	Donor	IVF:	In Vitro Fertilisation
S:	Surrogate mother	ET:	Embryo Transfer

extensive screening and only the most 'suitable' have any chance of adopting a healthy baby. There are still many thousands of older children available for fostering or adoption, and in need of loving homes. But many have social or emotional problems, or moderate to severe handicaps – and their needs are very special. The great majority are adopted by families who have already had children, feel confident as parents and perhaps have had some experience of handicapped children, so that they know how rewarding caring for them can be. But most childless couples do not feel able to adopt these needy children.

These factors have all meant that most infertile couples feel under more pressure than ever before to have a child of their own and, at the same time, medical science is opening new doors for them. Others, denied such solutions, or having tried them without success, are increasingly turning to unconventional ones such as surrogate motherhood, about which there has been much universal debate.

It is worth noting that many of the couples who are undergoing fertility treatment or, indeed, contemplating other arrangements such as surrogate motherhood would rather adopt than undergo the tests, lengthy treatment and uncertainty involved. One study of women attending IVF clinics in Australia showed that 63 per cent would have adopted – and 39 per cent would even have adopted a baby from abroad – had healthy babies been available or inter-country adoption procedures easier. So let us now consider the treatments and in what sort of circumstances they may be worth undertaking.

IN VITRO FERTILISATION (IVF)

Of all the new treatments available, still, none has had so much impact as in vitro fertilisation or IVF, the so-called 'test-tube baby' treatment. This is a way of completely bypassing blocked Fallopian tubes in women whose ovaries are functioning normally and who have a healthy womb.

IVF is a lengthy process. First, the woman's menstrual cycle has to be controlled with drugs such as chlomiphene (see Chapter 2) to ensure that she will ovulate at the right time for treatment. Drugs are usually used to stimulate her ovaries to produce more eggs or superovulate. (The woman's hormone levels have to be carefully monitored by blood tests and often by ultrasound scanning.) This is done so that several eggs can be fertilised, increasing the chance of success. Also, more than one embryo may be transferred, to increase the chance of at least one implanting and developing further.

The woman then goes into hospital for an egg retrieval operation, which involves a general anaesthetic. A gas is pumped into her abdomen and an instrument called a laparoscope is introduced through a small incision in her abdomen to view the ovaries and to remove any ripe eggs from the follicles. The retrieved eggs are kept in a special culture fluid to allow them to mature, then they are fertilised with the husband's sperm, which he is expected to produce by masturbation. Fresh semen is used if possible, as this increases the chance of success slightly, but under the stress of the procedure some men are unable to produce any. For this reason, sometimes semen is collected earlier and frozen in readiness for use at the appropriate time.

The sperm and eggs are mixed in the special culture solution to aid fertilisation. If it does take place, the embryos are allowed to develop for two to three days, to enable doctors to check that the development is normal. The embryos are then introduced into the woman's womb in a process usually referred to as embryo transfer. When the eggs are ready to be transferred, the woman usually receives injections of progesterone to prepare her womb. She will have to lie on her back with legs raised while the doctor passes a sterile catheter containing the culture fluid and embryos through the cervix (neck of the womb). A mild sedative may be given to help the woman relax during this procedure, as passing anything through the cervix can be quite uncomfortable. Following the transfer, most women are asked to rest in bed for a few hours before leaving the clinic.

If there is a choice of good embryos available, only the best will be introduced; if not, some embryos which appear less suitable may be used, as they do sometimes develop normally and produce a healthy baby. Most abnormal embryos are lost very early; there is no evidence that babies born through IVF are any more likely to be abnormal than those conceived naturally.

Success rate

So far, the success rate is only around 17 – 30 per cent. Many couples come back for at least three attempts; after this the success rate seems to fall even further, though some couples do finally succeed. Often, the embryo or embryos do not implant. Even if they do, early miscarriages can occur. About 30 per cent of IVF pregnancies miscarry as compared with about 10 per cent in the fertile population, for reasons which are not fully understood.

Over a period of months or years, attempts to conceive with the help of IVF can take over a couple's life. For the woman, it can be very difficult to keep a job or do anything else while IVF is being attempted. The frequent disappointments can seem overwhelming.

Many mothers also find that the existence of IVF makes it harder to 'let go' and accept their childlessness, or, if they already have one child, that their child will never have a brother or sister. This was the case with Sue.

Sue's story

'I had my first child without difficulty and never imagined any problems. When Joshua was two years and two months old we decided to try for a second. I became pregnant again quite soon but then started to bleed a lot and had agonising pain. I was rushed into hospital where they operated and found an ectopic pregnancy.

'I still had one tube, but when I conceived again the same thing happened. The consultant told me it might have happened because I had my appendix removed when I was pregnant with Joshua and that might have damaged the tubes. I was also told – very nicely – that I could never have any more children naturally but that there was hope with IVF.

'I have since tried twice through a private clinic. The second time I did get pregnant but miscarried at six weeks. I'm going to have one more try in October but we can't really afford any more treatment if that fails. There has to be a point where you call a halt. In some ways the existence of IVF makes it more difficult to give up. You think, one day we may be able to afford yet another try – there's always a ray of hope.'

Sadly, Sue's third attempt at IVF also failed to produce a pregnancy.

Jan and Len's story

In one of the early IVF success stories in Australia, Jan and Len did succeed, but with difficulties. Jan was infertile because she had suffered a severe infection in her Fallopian tubes. The couple's only hope was IVF.

In the first attempt, for some reason, fertilisation did not take place. The second time, an egg was fertilised and introduced into Jan's womb, but did not implant and early pregnancy tests were negative. The third time, two eggs were fertilised and transferred to her womb. This time pregnancy tests were positive; Jan was pregnant – with twins.

However, the problems were not over. At eight weeks of pregnancy, Jan began to bleed. She went into hospital where she was told one twin had been lost. Deeply distressed but comforted by the thought that one of her babies was still safe, Jan rested and then returned home. At fourteen weeks she began to bleed again, and returned to hospital. Fortunately, this time it was a false alarm and the pregnancy continued normally, resulting in a healthy 7lb baby girl.

GAMETE INTRA-FALLOPIAN TRANSFER (GIFT)

This technique uses much of the same technology as IVF. The eggs and sperm are collected as for IVF but then together re-introduced into the Fallopian tube, via the womb, in a similar process to embryo transfer with IVF, where it is hoped that fertilisation will occur naturally. GIFT is based on the possibility that, for some couples, the egg or sperm are failing to arrive at the site in the tubes where fertilisation is most likely to occur.

GIFT has had a success rate of 25 – 30 per cent, but can be used only where a woman has at least one normal Fallopian tube. It has also been used in cases where, despite extensive tests, no cause for a couple's infertility has been found. It can also help when the man has problems with his sperm – perhaps there are too few normal sperm to make the long journey into the Fallopian tubes or the woman's vagina or cervix may be hostile to sperm, making them unable to reach the womb. Although GIFT does bypass one whole phase of the full IVF programme, it is not much cheaper or less invasive to the couple.

ZYGOTE INTRA-FALLOPIAN TRANSFER (ZIFT)

In this variation of GIFT, the egg is transferred after fertilisation but before it divides.

TUBAL EMBRYO STAGE TRANSFER (TEST)

The embryos are transferred to the tubes rather than the womb as in standard IVF.

PERITONEAL OVUM AND SPERM TRANSFER (POST)

Again, this technique may be particularly helpful in cases where the man has poor sperm or the woman's vagina or cervix are hostile. It can be done without a general anaesthetic and as an out-patient procedure, unlike GIFT and IVF. The woman's eggs are collected in a syringe introduced through the abdominal wall. Then, together with the male partner's sperm already in the syringe, they are introduced into the abdomen near to the open ends of the Fallopian tubes, into which they are drawn. Fertilisation can then take place in the normal way.

Some specialists are afraid, however, that there might be an increased risk of ectopic pregnancy when this technique is used.

DIRECT INTRA-PERITONEAL INSEMINATION (DIPI)

DIPI is a a variation on this where washed sperm are placed in the Pouch of Douglas, an area between the womb and rectum into which eggs are believed to be shed when they are released from the ovary. The sperm are introduced via a needle inserted through the rear of the vagina.

Neither POST nor DIPI require a laparoscopy and are therefore cheaper and less risky to the potential mother.

However, direct intra-uterine insemination, when the woman's cycle has been stimulated by hormones, seems equally successful. Eggs and sperm can also be replaced together directly into the womb.

PROBLEMS WITH THE NEW TECHNIQUES

The techniques described above offer hope for many couples previously unable to have children. However, they also bring with them certain problems.

The technique of IVF in itself is not so controversial, though to many, the fertilisation of an egg outside the human body seems alarming, especially to those who believe that the embyro acquires the status of a human being from the moment of fertilisation. However, it is now usual for a woman receiving IVF to be treated with drugs which cause her to produce more than one egg. These may all then be fertilised, creating 'spare' embryos whose future is uncertain:

- They can be used to increase the woman's chance of a successful pregnancy by implanting several embryos at once.
- They can be frozen and stored for future use.
- They could be used for embryo research.
- They could be donated to another woman unable to produce her own eggs.

Early in the practise of IVF it was discovered that implanting several embryos into the womb could considerably increase the chance of at least one growing. Two, three, or four embryos are often implanted into a woman's womb. Usually, some of these embryos will be reabsorbed by the body, but not always; multiple pregnancies have often resulted. Many infertile couples are delighted to have twins, not least because their family is complete without the need for further treatment. But triplets or more can present problems, especially as the chances of the babies being miscarried, born premature or dying are considerably higher in multiple births.

If too many embryos do implant, it is possible to surgically destroy some of them. This is known as 'selective abortion' or 'foetal reduction'. What happens is that a drug – usually potassium chloride – is injected into the amniotic sac of the selected foetus, and the foetus is then absorbed into the mother's body. The procedure can be carried out as early as the ninth week of pregnancy, and is controlled by ultrasound, which enables the doctors to see the embryos on a screen. The procedure was originally developed for use where one of the embryos is handicapped, as diagnosed by tests in early pregnancy.

The procedure is highly controversial and it is not clear whether it should fall within legislation such as the British 1967 Abortion Act or not. Some doctors claim that because the pregnancy is not terminated and the foetus not expelled from the body, it cannot be described as an abortion.

Some doctors have implanted as many as seven embryos into the womb and then used foetal reduction, if necessary, to bring the number down to manageable levels. This use of the procedure has met with much opposition, although some women believe it offers them their only hope of parenthood. Others have had pregnancies reduced from two to one because they were at risk of having a miscarriage.

Many doctors feel that this practise of implanting more than four eggs knowing that, if too may 'take', some can be destroyed is unethical. However, even if a maximum of four embryos is used, it could result in quads, and this too could lead to problems, and perhaps the tragic loss of all four babies. The case of Mrs Jean Halton who gave birth to premature septuplets after fertility drug treatment, and then had to watch helplessly as each in turn died in the days and weeks after the birth, made the public and infertility patients painfully aware of the potential tragedy of multiple births.

Other would-be parents feel that, even if their triplets, quads or quins survived, they personally would not be able to cope.

'Because it has taken us so long and we've spent so many years having infertility tests and treatments, we're now quite old,' says Yvonne, who is 39 and whose husband is 45. 'I could cope with twins – with a bit of help – but how would I cope with three or more? How would we give them the attention they need? So we feel torn. On the one hand we know, as we've so little time left, that the chances of a successful pregnancy are much greater if they implant more eggs. On the other hand, if we had a multiple pregnancy, we might lose all the babies and even if we didn't, we wouldn't know how to cope.'

Some mothers, not offered foetal reduction, have even decided on complete termination of the pregnancy because they were expecting quads. This must be the ultimate tragedy: to take desperate measures to have a baby, and then have to terminate a pregnancy because they are carrying too many.

Foetal reduction itself is not without risks. One clinic recently reported that in about half of the cases where selective reduction was used, all the foetuses were lost. One British woman who had five embryos take after IVF chose to have three teminated. The operation resulted in the loss of all five. In *The Guardian* newspaper of 23 July 1987 she wrote: 'It was like the end of everything. Being infertile was pretty awful. But this time I felt I had deliberately destroyed life I had created. I had been greedy and I was punished for my greed. It was my decision. The doctor explained the risks ... I won't try again.'

DONOR EGGS

'Ordinary' IVF may help a woman to conceive if she is producing healthy eggs but has blocked tubes. What happens, however, if she does not produce eggs? A new option possible as a spin-off from IVF is that she could receive a donor egg. This can be accomplished in two ways:

- Donor eggs can be collected from another woman by laparoscopy, as for IVF, and then fertilised with the infertile woman's partner's sperm. The embryo can then be implanted into her womb.
- The husband's sperm can be used to inseminate the woman donating the egg, and the egg is then fertilised normally in her body. The fertilised egg is then flushed out of the donor's womb in a technique called 'lavage' and implanted into the receiving womb. Certain risks are attached to lavage: the fertilised egg can be washed into a Fallopian tube and cause an ectopic pregnancy, or the egg can be left behind leaving the 'donor' pregnant, or an infection can be introduced. For these reasons the technique is not used at present.

Because the act of giving an egg involves a considerable degree of involvement – the egg donor may need treatment with fertility drugs to induce her to produce more then one egg and she has to undergo the minor surgery of a laparoscopy – it is unlikely that there would be as many casual egg donors as there might be sperm donors. The most likely candidates are women already undergoing infertility treatments who perhaps produce more eggs than they need. However, these mothers might be older women or in other ways not ideal to act as donors. Also, it would not be possible to match donors with recipients for similar characteristics as it is with sperm donors.

The first pregnancy achieved with a donor egg was carried out in Australia, using the egg of a 42-year-old infertility patient simply because she happened to be there at the time. The pregnancy miscarried at ten weeks and the foetus was found to have a chromosomal abnormality, much more common in older women. Using this woman as donor was criticised by other doctors involved in IVF as being irresponsible.

Close relatives as donors

Those most likely to act as egg donors are close friends and relatives of the infertile couple. Most cases of egg donation have so far involved friends or sisters. Some have been arranged between mother and daughter or aunt and niece, but in such cases the donor's egg might then be fertilised by her father or uncle – relationships considered incestuous in law.

Apart from considerations of incest, many doctors and others fear that it could cause confusion for the child and possibly family tensions. A woman who had given birth to a baby for her sister, for example, might disapprove of something the mother was doing in bringing up the child. She might then be tempted to interfere and thus put pressure on the mother or child. If family relations broke down, the child might be presented with two well-loved figures each claiming to be his or her 'real' mother.

Despite such apparent pitfalls, many people still see using a close relative's egg or sperm as preferable to that of an unknown donor. A story which appeared in the press in 1983 concerned a couple who were unable to have children because the wife was infertile. She had a sister to whom she was very close, who had two children of her own and enjoyed pregnancy and motherhood.

The infertile couple obtained an insemination cap from a private clinic, ostensibly to help conception, but the husband used this to inseminate his wife's sister, who conceived and gave birth to his child. Soon after the birth she handed over the baby to her sister and the baby's father to bring up as their child. For the infertile sister, the baby born of her sister and husband was as close as possible genetically to the child she might herself have had had she been fertile. In the United States, a similar story involved identical twin sisters, which meant the child born was genetically identical to the one the infertile sister would have had.

More recent cases have involved the donation of an egg by one sister to another who was unable to ovulate normally. The first babies, twins, to be born by this technique were born six weeks prematurely at a hospital in the north of England with no publicity, because everyone believed they were the result of ordinary IVF. The mother originally planned to use an anonymous egg donor, but one could not be found. Her older sister had completed her own family, so was hoping to donate an egg. Neither sister believes there is a problem. 'I feel that they are my children – they grew inside me after all,' says the twin's mother, while her sister says, 'I regard the babies as totally my sister's children.'

Another case was that of Nora Cherriman, who was born with a rare condition called ovarian dysgenesis, which means that her ovaries never existed. At the age of 30 she was finally made pregnant with her sister's egg, fertilised with her husband Garry's sperm. Nora said: 'We would not have been happy to use eggs from a donor we knew nothing about – nothing about their history or their life. We chose Theresa because we are close in age, and we look alike. And with my sister's eggs we are continuing the family's bloodline – at least there is still that connection with my parents and grandparents.'

Robin and Simon Ooi are Chinese twins born from frozen

embryos conceived from their father's sperm and their aunt's eggs in the ultimate high technology birth. Their birth overcame years of anguish and created great happiness for the whole extended family.

Susie Ooi had had cysts removed from her ovaries at the age of 23. After attempts to have a child naturally and a course of hormone treatment which failed, she was told she was infertile. In addition, she then had to face the trauma of a premature menopause. She tried adoption agencies who said they had a two-year waiting list and that anyway, no Chinese babies were available. Then Dr Simon Fishel at AMI Park Hospital, Nottingham, who had heard about her case, offered her IVF with donor eggs.

Susie's sister, Carol, who had four healthy children in Malaysia, agreed to have three laparoscopies to remove a total of six eggs which were fertilised by Susie's husband John's sperm. Three fresh embryos were implanted into her womb and the other three were frozen and stored. Susie, who had received hormone treatment to prepare her body for pregnancy, found to her delight that she was pregnant, but she miscarried within four weeks. The frozen embryos were then thawed, observed to check that they were growing normally and implanted. The pregnancy took and twin boys were born 10 weeks premature, but healthy.

'One day we will tell them of their conception,' says Susie, 'They have a right to know. I believe they will be happy to know what greatly wanted children they are.' She also believes a sister makes the best donor; 'It would be the closest thing to my own baby. There would be no sense of wondering where certain characteristics come from. I mean, look at Simon – he looks like my own side of the family while Robin looks like John.'

Others involved in sister-to-sister egg donation have said that they would not want to tell their children. Some had even kept it secret from parents and other relatives, partly because they feel there is 'no need to tell' but also perhaps because they fear the possible confusion caused to the child.

However, many people have been adopted by sisters or brothers and there is no particular evidence to show that this has been more problematic for them than being adopted by strangers. In fact, there is evidence that fostering by relatives is more successful than fostering by strangers (see Chapter 7).

SURROGATE MOTHERHOOD

If a woman is unable to carry a baby in her womb – she may have a congenital abnormality of the uterus or had to have a hysterectomy – she may consider the age-old option of surrogate motherhood. The Bible tells of more than one incident where, when a woman was unable to conceive, her husband conceived a child with a servant girl. The story of Rachel is perhaps the best known.

Today surrogate motherhood is mainly practised in the United States where commercial agencies pay the surrogate mother for conceiving and carrying the baby and then handing it over at birth to the commissioning parents. In Britain commercial surrogacy is illegal, but surrogacy arrangements are still carried out, often with money changing hands 'under the counter'.

Surrogate motherhood is probably the most complex of all arrangements made to enable an infertile couple to have children. In fact there are two kinds of surrogacy:

- 'Full surrogacy', where a surrogate mother is the genetic mother of the child she carries, having conceived with the sperm of the infertile woman's partner.
- 'Partial surrogacy', or using a 'host mother', where the commissioning mother's egg is fertilised with her partner's sperm and then implanted into another woman's womb. This requires medical intervention, so is more difficult to achieve, though many couples would prefer it if it were possible. This technique has also been called 'renting a womb' by the popular press.

Possible problems

The main problem with surrogacy of both kinds is that the woman who carried and gave birth to the child may find herself, in the end, unable to part with the baby. This is more likely when the baby is genetically hers. Although most arrangements seem to go ahead without great trauma, some surrogate mothers have regretted their involvement and come out publicly against it. America's first surrogate mother recently told the world's press that she had come to long for the child she gave away.

Surrogacy is quite common now in the United States; there are over 20 surrogate parenthood organisations and by the end of 1983 they claimed to have been responsible for over 500 births. Though most of these contracts have been carried out without any problems, those that have not show the potential minefield that surrogate arrangements can become.

Some case histories

One of the worst stories took place in the United States in 1983/1984. A couple commissioned a Mrs Stiver to give birth to a baby. When the baby was born it was severely handicapped. The 'father', Mr Malahoff, decided he did not want the baby and denied that the child was his. Blood tests were taken, and it turned out that this was indeed the case – Mrs Stiver had not been told not to have sex with her husband at the time of the insemination.

Mr Malahoff then sued Mrs Stiver for not producing the child he commissioned. The Stivers sued those responsible in the surrogate organisation for not giving them proper instructions and sued Mr Malahoff for violating their privacy by making the story public. They also claimed that the child was handicapped because of a virus present in Mr Malahoff's sperm.

Another case which received a great deal of publicity, was that of 'Baby M'. The commissioning parents, William and Elisabeth Stern, were a professional couple both aged 41. They wanted a baby, but Mrs Stern had diagnosed herself as suffering from multiple sclerosis and was afraid that a pregnancy would worsen her condition. They therefore commissioned Mary Beth Whitehead to have a baby for them.

When the baby was born, Mary Beth handed her over as planned. But soon she was back on the doorstep, begging them to give her the baby. The Sterns did so because they said they were afraid of what she might do to herself if they didn't carry out her wishes. They then began the fight to get the baby back. When the case was finally heard the judge decided to give custody of the child to the Sterns as he felt that they would make the best parents.

Mary Beth Whitehead was denied not only all parental rights but any access to the child. No-one had ever suggested that she was an unsuitable parent to her two sons, and no-one doubted her maternal feelings. But Judge Sorkow concluded that the surrogate parenting agreement is a valid and enforceable contract, and stressed the father's right to his own biological genetically related child.

In the event, however, this ruling was finally overturned by the New Jersey Supreme Court the following February, nearly two years after baby M's birth. The court ruled that surrogate contracts were illegal because the buying and selling of babies was illegal; it gave Mary Beth Whitehead regular visitation rights and revoked Elisabeth Stern's right to adopt the baby, which she had done as a step-parent, though the Sterns retained custody.

Some say that this ruling had not solved the problem and had left the child with a less certain future and with two mothers. It is difficult, in any event, to see who could come out of such a situation without pain, whatever the final ruling.

The Sterns' contract was arranged by lawyer Noel Keane of Dearborn, Michigan, an acknowleged pioneer of the surrogate baby business. He started in 1976 and had many successful cases before he gave up his general law practice and started the Infertility Centre in New York City. Keane finds the surrogate, arranges doctors' appointments for insemination, drafts legal papers, organises maternity hospital bookings and arranges a physical and psychological assessment of the surrogate.

Noel Keane encourages his infertile couples and the surrogates to become friends. While this can result in a happy outcome, it can result in the parties coming to dislike one another, and this may make it more difficult for the surrogate mother to part with the baby or the commissioning couple to totally accept the baby when it is born.

Another of Noel Keane's success stories involves Laura and

her husband, who ended up with two daughters four months apart after using two surrogates. She says: 'At first I felt great jealousy and resentment. After all, there was this younger woman being impregnated with my husband's sperm. It caused all sorts of feelings inside me and although I tried to hide them, as my husband wanted a baby of his own so badly, I really didn't want him to see the pictures of the surrogates at first – I was so jealous. Then Noel suggested we meet one of them and that actually made me feel a lot better, as I realised that she didn't want anything to do with my husband. Because of course, that was what had been bothering me.'

Other agencies such as that of Harriet Blankfield, responsible for Kim Cotton's surrogate baby in Britain, keeps the identities of the surrogate and the commissioning couple separate from one another. One surrogate mother for Harriet Blankfield, Kyle Adams, confessed that 'If I knew the identity of the couple, then in years to come I might be tempted to drive down the street where they live to see whether there is a little boy playing in their driveway.' During her pregnancy, Kyle Adams wrote to the couple, giving them a lot of information about herself but receiving little in return. The birth was complicated and resulted in a Caesarian section, and the new parents came to take the baby from the hospital while Kyle was still feeling groggy after the operation – they did not leave her a note or send her flowers. Understandably she felt bitter about this treatment.

Noel Keane's agency was responsible for 175 of the estimated 500 surrogate babies now born in the US. He tells of many happy outcomes where parents and surrogates remain friends. One woman wrote of the surrogate, 'Debbie was special and always will be. We did become friends and shared the joy of her pregnancy and birth. I miss talking to her, but I know it's best not to continue a close relationship.' Another surrogate mother recalls: 'We wanted to keep in touch and a really close relationship has developed, even though the couple live far away in Canada. The couple and I kept in constant touch (throughout the pregnancy) and I shared everything with them. I never lost sight of the fact that it was their baby.'

The surrogates and their families

While people have considered the problems for the surrogate mother, few have thought of her family. The ideal surrogate is seen as a married woman who has completed her own family. But what do her children think when their mother gives away the new baby to strangers, never to be seen again? Some psychiatrists have predicted that these children will suffer fear of being given away themselves. If mother gave away one baby for money, might she not be tempted to do the same with them . . .

What *are* the motives of women willing to go through a pregnancy and birth and then give up the baby, perhaps never to see the child again? Clearly the motives are usually more than purely commercial, as summed up in the title of British surrogate mother Kim Cotton's book, *Baby Cotton – For Love and Money*.

The motives of surrogate mothers are clearly mixed, depending on their relationship to the infertile couple. Women who have had particular insight into the problems of the infertile may see having a baby for another couple as a worthwhile thing. Sometimes close friends or relatives of an infertile woman offer to have her baby. Where the mothers have been strangers, approached through an agency or advertisement, they talk of a mixture of a desire to do something they are good at to both earn money to improve their own life and to help an infertile couple.

The published stories of two women unrelated to the parents-to-be who became surrogate mothers show that they were also seeking some kind of emotional gratification from the experience and that in this, both were disappointed.

'Kirsty Stevens' (a pseudonym) in her book *Surrogate Mother: One Woman's Story* shows her disappointment and bitterness that the hoped-for intimacy with Robert and Jean, the couple she had a child for, failed to materialise. 'I had been looking forward to having womanly chats over the telephone, and instead it was . . . Robert acting as a go-between, and Jean and me never talking to each other directly . . . the friendly calls I had been expecting never came.'

She concluded '. . . I felt totally empty. For the first time I started thinking that Robert and Jean had used me. That feeling has persisted.'

'Kirsty Stevens' was very naive in expecting that the parents of her baby might want to go on knowing her – in many ways, she was an embarrassment to them, a reminder that the child was not entirely 'theirs'. She may also have seemed a threat, especially as someone who so obviously sought a close relationship, someone who seemed emotionally needy.

Kim Cotton, whose baby was conceived and brought into the world for another couple on 4 January 1985, brought a storm of publicity about surrogacy in Britain, also wrote in her book, *Baby Cotton – For Love and Money*, of feelings of rejection:

'It hurt me terribly to know that they might hate me. I would have loved it if they had written to me, care of the solicitor, to say they didn't blame me (for the baby being made a ward of court after the birth and all the publicity) and that they loved the baby.' She was also very sad that she had not heard how the parents had reacted to their new baby. 'I wanted to know everything . . . What did they think of the baby? Who held her first? Who said what?'

Again, Kim Cotton was seeking emotional gratification through what she had done. When she did not receive it, she felt wounded and let down. Although she still supports the need for surrogate motherhood, she admitted to a national newspaper in January 1986; 'I got a lot more pain than I ever thought I would . . .'.

Clearly the time after the birth is a difficult one for all surrogate mothers. 'Kirsty Stevens' writes of the difficulty she experienced dealing with her own maternal feelings: 'Apart from my disappointment over Robert and Jean, my greatest difficulty during those first months was not having anything on which to focus my strong maternal feelings. Once I left Alan (the baby) behind I thought I would be able somehow to transfer the feelings on to my own boys. But the boys are too old for that now: they didn't want it.

'I began feeling broody again. This took me by surprise: I hadn't at all intended to have another baby yet . . . For four months or so, I was very keen to get pregnant again. (But) when it didn't happen immediately my strong feelings began to subside . . . Gradually they more or less disappeared.'

In other cases, the surrogate mother and the couple do manage to remain friends. Mary Stewart answered an adver-

tisement (now illegal) in the local paper reading
'SURROGATE mother wanted for childless couple'. She
conceived and gave birth to a son for Gena and Mike Dodd
(see Chapter 3). Mary and Gena agreed to keep in touch with
one another every week until the baby, John, was three years
old. Gena writes 'Mike didn't like the idea and he said it never
gave Mary a chance to forget and build a new life for herself.
Once John could be told how and why he was born, he could
make up his own mind if he wanted the relationship to carry
on.'

Gena Dodd said she did not feel jealousy in her relationship
with the surrogate, Mary, except briefly when her husband
slept with her to get her pregnant. They used what the couple
called 'the natural method' so that doctors would not be
involved ... clearly a very difficult process for all concerned.
Gena saw Mary regularly during the pregnancy and was
present during the birth.

'I never felt jealousy – I never felt it was Mary's baby. It's
a funny feeling, but I don't feel John as anything but mine.'

A remarkable surrogacy

When a woman closely related to a childless couple becomes
involved, the motives become different, though also complex.
Recently a 48-year-old South African woman, Pat Anthony,
made medical, social and legal history by giving birth to her
daughter's triplets, conceived through IVF.

Pat's daughter Karen had had a hysterectomy following
complications after the birth of her son. Desperate to have
another child, she tried to find a surrogate mother, without
success. Then Pat, who had given birth to two children herself,
offered to act as surrogate. Her daughter's eggs were fertilised
by her son-in-law's sperm and four embryos transferred to her
womb, resulting in a triplet pregnancy. The babies, two boys
and a girl, were all healthy.

The daughter, Karen, had hormone treatment to enable her
to breastfeed her babies after the birth. Legal custody was
given to Pat Anthony until the triplets' genetic parents adopted
them, which as close relatives, they could easily do. And Pat
Anthony will be able to watch the babies' development with a

special 'grandmotherly' pride, whereas so many surrogates –
as we have seen – lose sight of their child for ever.

The long-term effects

When we come to consider the long-term effects of giving up
the child, the experience of mothers who relinquished a child
for adoption are not very reassuring (see Chapter 7). The
feelings of surrogate mothers may be complicated by the fact
that while mothers who gave up their child for adoption usually
never intended a pregnancy, or got pregnant expecting to
marry the father, the surrogate may have had very complex
motives for her undertaking. In an article in the *Washington
Post*, Elizabeth Bumiller, a Michigan psychologist, claimed
that about one-third of applicants to be surrogate mothers may
participate in order to atone for previous abortions.

One study carried out by a US doctor looked at 30 women
who had been surrogates. All 30 were white, and aged from 19
to 33; 26 were married, 3 single and 1 divorced. Two had
never been pregnant before, 12 had either had an abortion or
given up a previous child for adoption. The women said they
became surrogates to earn money, to enjoy pregnancy, and
give the infertile couple the gift of a baby. Most of the women
felt content and pleased with the special attention they received
while being pregnant, and felt they were doing something
worthwhile.

Some of the women who had previously had an abortion or
given up a child said they felt being a surrogate had helped
them deal with prior feelings of loss – because they had chosen
to get pregnant and give away the child this time and felt more
in control.

The women had different ways of dealing with the fact they
were going to give the baby up; describing the child as 'theirs,
not mine', having contact with the eventual parents and ideal-
ising them as good parents, and seeing the process as a sharing
between them and the couple. One-third of the surrogates
formed a support group during their pregnancies and became
close friends.

The surrogate mothers' feelings on giving up the child were
varied. One mother had nightmares during the pregnancy that

the baby would be deformed and the couple wouldn't want it. One had nightmares about giving the baby up; another said she felt no sense of loss at all. Some had varying degrees of crying and sadness for several weeks. Some of the women said their sadness was linked to the loss of their relationship with the couple rather than the baby. Three sought psychiatric treatment or counselling to help them deal with the loss and one was briefly given anti-depressants. Some of them felt anger and resentment towards the couples after the birth because they got less attention than they had done before. Most of the women wondered how the baby would fare in future. Many wanted to be informed periodically of its progress, either directly or indirectly.

The report does not say how many of these mothers overlap; for example, whether the ones who were depressed after the birth were the same as those who wanted a replacement child or the same ones who had nightmares. However, it does show that there is a strong likelihood that the surrogate mother will suffer loss after the birth, and may need help in coming to terms with this.

This shows that the problems with having a surrogate baby are not over for either party even if the surrogate hands over the baby and is prepared to sign adoption papers. As the baby Cotton case showed, the social services can also intervene and make the child a ward of court or take other action. This is done with the intention of protecting the child, but can be very distressing for all concerned.

World views on surrogacy

The major reports on artificial reproduction commissioned by governments in the United Kingdom, Australia, Canada and New Zealand have all tried to address the problem of surrogate motherhood. All started off with the viewpoint that surrogate motherhood was undesirable, and sought ways to discourage the practice, while accepting that a small number of people were likely always to resort to it. The reports were chiefly concerned with preventing commercial surrogacy arrangements.

In the UK, the Warnock report suggested banning all commercial surrogacy arrangements and this piece of legislation was then enacted as the Surrogacy Arrangements Act in 1985. All legal contracts for surrogacy arrangements are invalid and unenforceable, and advertising for a surrogate mother is also illegal. Lawyers or doctors who tried to help set up a surrogacy arrangement would also be operating outside the law and could face prosecution, though this is unclear.

In Australia, Victoria's Infertility (Medical Procedures) Act of 1984 makes entry into a surrogate motherhood agreement punishable whether or not payment is involved. However, this does not cover surrogacy arrangements where natural intercourse is involved, and couples can use this – or claim to have used it – in order to evade the legislation.

In Canada, in 1985, the Ontario Law Reform Commission issued its Report on Human Artificial Reproduction and Related Matters. This took a fundamentally different attitude. While the commission did not seek to promote the practice it felt that the best interests of children born through surrogate arrangements must take precedence. It proposed a surrogate adoption procedure which would enable all parties in a surrogate motherhood agreement to seek approval from a Family Court judge. The agreement should be specifically enforceable, if need be by seizing the child from the surrogate mother if she refused to surrender it at birth. This would tend to discourage mothers in any doubt about whether they would be able to give up their child, and would help prevent mothers from keeping the baby in order to force the commissioning parents to pay her large (illegal) sums of money.

The problem of exploitation

There has been much discussion about the ethics of surrogate motherhood and whether it is a valuable service which one woman can provide for others, being paid for her services, or whether it is a form of exploitation or prostitution.

Carl Wood, the Australian IVF pioneer quoted in Susan Downie's 1988 book *Babymaking* seems to take the first view, claiming that surrogate motherhood can work and be 'one of the most generous, loving and humane acts that one woman can carry out for another'. He believes it might have wider benefits for society, too. 'It will teach us to see childbearing from a wider perspective than of two parents ... I am optimistic that skilled surrogacy could become one of the most successful infertility therapies. It has suffered from inadequate support and study, overexposure of the complications in the media and unfair prejudice.'

However, in practice things may be rather different. In a book entitled *Test-tube Women: What Future for Motherhood,* a collection of essays by various women, Susan Ince writes a first-hand account of applying to be a surrogate mother in the US. She reveals that the 'psychological interviews' seemed mostly aimed at seeing if she would do what she was told rather than looking into her medical/psychological history, how she would feel about carrying and giving birth to another man's child and whether she would feel able to give up the child. She discovered that anonymity would not be preserved because the father would see her name on the birth certificate and also have access to the baby in hospital and possibly at the birth.

She also points out that the mother will get no fee for a miscarried child or a baby aborted after an amniocentesis reveals it to be abnormal. This is open to abuse, as there is no protection for the surrogate should the parents opt for an abortion if the baby is the 'wrong sex'. There is no compensation if the mother becomes ill as a result of pregnancy or birth. If the surrogate decides to keep the child the parents may sue her for the $25,000 fee they paid to the programme plus additional costs. If the parents refuse to take the child or pay the surrogate's medical expenses, the mother may sue them, but won't get any support from the agency.

Susan Ince argues that it is the father who commissions the child and for whom the surrogate is working – this is like prostitution, and the lawyers, doctors or others who employ the surrogate and commission the couples are like pimps. It is also possible that in some surrogate arrangements the father is pushing ahead with it to have his 'own' child while the infertile wife might prefer some other solution to their infertility. In some cases single men have used surrogates to have their child.

Susan Ince argues that even if you view the surrogate mother as a self-employed person, she is liable to exploitation and should be protected. The majority of surrogate mothers are likely to be poor and unskilled, working for rich professional couples. Further, for most surrogates at the moment there is no follow-up or counselling to help them deal with emotional problems in pregnancy or their feelings on giving the child up after the birth.

The fact that commercial surrogacy seems to exploit the surrogate mother led to its being banned in Britain under the Surrogacy Arrangements Act 1985.

Professional opinions

Many infertility specialists believe that there *is* a limited place for surrogacy – if it could be provided as part of an infertility programme, following suitable counselling, protection for the surrogate and adequate follow-up. Robert Winston of the Hammersmith Hospital, London, in his book, *Infertility: a Sympathetic Approach*, writes: 'Despite my very grave reservations regarding every aspect of surrogacy, I admit that there are certain very rare situations in which it may be a perfectly reasonable option.'

In fact, surrogacy is a very effective fertility treatment – much more likely to succeed than IVF – and provided the couple and the surrogate were counselled, potential problems could be avoided. Even if it were accepted that the surrogate mother could keep the baby if she chose, and that she retained that right till signing adoption papers, this would be a small risk that the couple would have to take on board, similar to the risk of their baby being miscarried or stillborn.

ARTIFICIAL INSEMINATION BY DONOR (AID)

When a man is found to be infertile, AID at present offers the only solution to the majority of couples desperate to have a baby. It is estimated that between two and three thousand children are born every year in Britain through AID, and thousands more every year in the USA. AID simply means that a woman receives the sperm of an unknown donor, placed in her vagina by a medical practitioner, in a simple procedure in which a tube is inserted into the vagina to deliver sperm near to the cervix. Strictly speaking, a medical practitioner is not really necessary. Couples can, and have, chosen a friend as donor and used an insemination cap, contraceptive cap or syringe to introduce the sperm into the woman's vagina.

With the advent of the disease AIDS (auto-immune deficiency syndrome), however, most people would want to know that the donor has been medically screened to make sure he is not suffering from any disease. Screening should also ensure that the donor's sperm are plentiful and normal and that the woman therefore stands a good chance of getting pregnant.

AID was available to a few as early as the 1930s and some gynaecologists used AID during the war, where it seemed the only solution to male infertility. In 1945 the first full account of AID was published in the *British Medical Journal*, and provoked public controversy. The issue was later debated in Parliament and the Feversham Committee was appointed; its report, published in 1960, concluded that AID was undesirable.

However, AID continued to be practised and changing attitudes towards many sexual matters, together with a decline in the number of children available for adoption, eventually ensured that AID became more acceptable to a growing number of infertile couples.

In 1970 the British Medical Association appointed a panel of inquiry under Sir John Peel and its report, published in 1973, was more favourable. But the status of AID is still not clear. Children born through AID are technically illegitimate, and should be registered at birth with 'father unknown.' The couple can then arrange for the social father to adopt the child. In practise the baby is usually registered as the couple's own. This means that secrecy and deception are practised on a large scale, making any follow-up of AID children more difficult, and denying the child an automatic right to know about his or her origins.

Studies have shown that the vast majority of AID couples have no intention of telling their children. Robert Snowden's interviews with almost 70 couples with AID children (published in the book he wrote with Elizabeth Snowden, *The Gift of a Child*) showed that while almost all intended not to tell the children, 40 per cent had confided in other people, including members of the family. For an Australian study by Robyn Rowland, published in 1985, 93 couples in an AID programme were interviewed and it was found that only 9 per cent intended to tell the children. Of the remainder, 56 per cent planned not to tell and 35 per cent were unsure. Again, though, a high proportion of these couples had told someone else. Only 36 per cent said they had told no-one.

The couples concerned did not seem to have considered that the children might one day find out through relatives or friends who had been let into the secret, although it is fairly widely known that, in the case of adoption, other people often *do* tell the children, sometimes after the parent's death when there is no opportunity ever to discuss it with them. Indeed, many couples had not anticipated that not telling might become increasingly difficult as the child got older. The motives for not telling are also interesting.

Motives for secrecy

Many parents do not tell because they feel uncomfortable about admitting to the father's infertility. Many people still consider that a man who is infertile must be sexually inadequate and this can cause the man in question to conceal his problem from all but those he is most intimate with. In such circumstances, the couple may fear that if the child knows, he or she may tell others. Couples may also fear that the paternal grandparents – if they knew – might have difficulties in relating to the child who is not related to them by blood.

Some couples do not tell because they do not know how to explain to the child about AID. By the time the child is old enough to understand, it may seem less and less easy to tell, and when the child is an adolescent the normal tensions between parents and children may make it even more problematical. The longer the secret is kept, the more difficult it is to bring it out into the open. As one husband quoted in the Snowdens' book, *The Gift of a Child*, explained: ' . . . you start a deceit or pretence right at the start and you have got to maintain it. It is like any white lie or lies, it snowballs . . . You know in your heart that you haven't told anyone the truth.'

One wife said 'I think if we had told them (the grandparents) straightaway perhaps they wouldn't have minded; but now I think they would think "Why couldn't they have told us earlier?"'.

The stress of secrecy

Some parents find that they are constantly caught out. One woman, for example, was constantly drawn by friends into discussions about which contraceptives they were using, which she found hard to deal with. Another felt anxious because most people knew what problems she and her husband had had in having a baby and she wondered if they had guessed at the solution. Children, too, are often very perceptive and may guess at the truth, as Clare did:

'I was adopted because my parents couldn't have any children. Then, a few years later, my mother was suddenly pregnant. One day she was telling me about the facts of life and she also told me about AID. I remember thinking how odd it was at the time, especially as she went into so much detail. It just didn't seem relevant.

'My sister and I didn't get on very well. I suppose I was jealous because she was my parent's "real" child, though oddly, I never felt she had any connection with my father. She didn't look like him or anything. Years later it came to me in a flash, "I wonder if they used AID'. It made everything make sense, though I've never dared to ask my mother, and I don't think that my sister knows; if she does, she's never mentioned it to me.'

Fear of being found out may cast a cloud over the couple's happiness with their child in ways they might not have imagined. Those who are open feel much more relaxed about it. Almost all find that family and friends react positively to the news. Many grandparents, in particular, want their children to have a child as much or more than the parents do. Some grandparents may be a little apprehensive or shocked at first, but almost all seem to accept the child once it is born.

Children's reaction

If the children are told, how do they react? Many told when they are young adults seem to accept their AID status without problems. One young man said that his acceptance of the news had even surprised himself. A young girl felt that her parents must have wanted her very much to go through all the problems of treatment. 'They must love me a tremendous amount, and realising that makes me love them even more, too.'

Some children suspect that something is 'odd', as we saw in the case of Clare, and may find the news a relief from their doubts. One girl explained, 'Being told made me feel as if a huge great weight had been lifted off my shoulders.'

Where secrecy has been maintained, the knowledge of AID can come about in unfortunate circumstances. One child was told by her mother as her parents divorced: 'Of course, you were never his child in the first place.' Such children may find this revelation a terrible blow, as they may feel they have lost their father twice over.

Another child, told after her father's death, recalls bitterly, 'I wish I had been able to talk to him about it. If only I had been able to tell him that I didn't care about AID, that to me he always was and always will be my father.'

Perhaps more tragic is the story of Suzanne Rubin, who found out about her AID origins only when she was over 30 and her mother had died. Suzanne had always thought there was something odd about her parents and herself: her parents were Jewish, with black hair and brown and grey eyes; she was red-haired and blue eyed. When she was seven she heard about adoption and began to search the house for papers. At 15 she became pregnant and gave up the baby for adoption. After her mother died of cancer when Suzanne was 29, she began a search for her daughter, and located her after six months. The reunion was not a joyous one, but at least Suzanne felt she had given her her history.

Suzanne's father opposed her search for her daughter and finally broke down and told her about her AID origins. She wanted to know who the donor was but her father could only say he didn't know, but the practitioner had told him the donor was Jewish. Suzanne knew most donors were medical students so she traced the 55 Jewish medical students in the hospital in the year of her conception but some of them told her to look for the doctor who had carried out the inseminations. When she saw a photograph of him, she knew at once that he was her father.

Suzanne felt that not only she but her parents had been deceived. She has considered taking the doctor to court, not to hurt him, but to change the system and protect the rights of other AID children.

In a letter to the editor of a school paper at an earlier date, she wrote an indictment of the practice of AID: 'Artificial insemination sounds wonderful in the textbooks, but what it can do to human lives is something else. By encouraging very young, very immature and very short-sighted males to become sperm donors, you are creating countless triads of husband and wife and donor. Unfortunately the missing component is the child. No one considers how the child feels when she finds that her father was a $25 cup of sperm. The fantasies revolve around what the donor was thinking of when he filled the cup.

'There is no passion, no human contact in such a union; just cold calculation and manipulation of another person's life. And for those of you who feel that a healthy family relationship can be built around a foundation of deliberate lies, I would wonder what fantasy life you have been living in.'

Suzanne Rubin's story is alarming because there are so many doctors practising AID, especially in the United States, without any kind of regulation or control. The kind of deception that she experienced may not be uncommon.

Need for counselling

Almost all the medical studies of AID are positive about the outcome, but the issue is very complex and problems might be deepfelt. Consequently, more and more doctors and infertility counsellors feel that it is vital for couples considering AID to receive counselling and raise any hidden fears.

Some wives fantasise about the donor, especially before the baby is born, perhaps imagining him as a 'perfect man' in the image of a film star or other fantasy figure or alternatively fearing that he might be a criminal or even a murderer.

One study of 50 couples who had had AID children, carried out by Christine Clayton and Gabor Kovacs in Melbourne, published in 1982, showed that all wives were anxious about their husbands' reaction to the child before the birth and four described problems in the husband's relationship with the child. One husband felt that the child was a constant reminder of his infertility.

In fact, it is not uncommon for husbands to feel inadequate in the face of the donors who got their partners pregnant when they could not. Some AID fathers experience painful jealousy, especially during their wife's pregnancy. Others find themselves hating the doctor.

One man's account of how AID, carried out without proper counselling, nearly destroyed his marriage, his self-esteem and his relationship with his two children is chillingly told in his book *Blizzard and the Holy Ghost*.

A retrospective study of one AID counsellor's case records at the Royal Women's Hospital Melbourne during 1981 showed that at the first interview 18 out of the 50 couples recognised that one or both partners were not ready to accept AID, despite having previously informed doctors that they wished to proceed. These couples needed further counselling over a period of months to deal with marital, sexual and interpersonal problems before achieving a genuinely positive motivation for AID. Two couples decided to withdraw in recognition of their inability to accept AID.

This counsellor, Jenny Hunt – now working as an infertility counsellor at the Hammersmith Hospital London – says that the necessity for careful counselling is brought home to her by the couples she sees who have attended other AID programmes where they have only had brief communication with the doctor.

- Many of these couples do not understand basic facts about AID and report emotional traumas and marital difficulties.
- Some women are repelled by the act of insemination.
- Some are confused about the selection of donors, and many say they had no-one to turn to.
- It still seems common practice for doctors to advise secrecy, and this may compound some people's sense of guilt, isolation and fear.

At the Hammersmith Hospital, couples considering AID are counselled first together, then separately, then together again. This allows them to express their fears and hopes first separately, and then together. Some couples have doubts which they feel unable to express to their partner for fear of causing pain, but find it helpful to raise these with a counsellor. This may then enable them to talk more openly among one another.

If these issues are not dealt with in the beginning, problems can fester for years. There is no evidence that marriages where AID has occurred are any less stable than other marriages, but where they do break up, AID may be a complicating factor. Sometimes, indeed, it may be the cause.

One AID parent whose marriage later broke up originally agreed to his wife having artificial insemination primarily for her sake, but when the child was born he became just as emotionally involved, and still is. 'Since the separation however, I am not allowed to see my child . . . my wife has told me I am only her guardian.'

The donor

One member of the AID triangle who is often dismissed is the donor. People have long been suspicious of the donor's motives; most have been young medical students, giving sperm to make a little extra money. The ethics of giving payment for donating sperm has been debated, but the practice still continues. In some countries, however – for example France – the donor must be a married man who already has children and must not be paid for his services.

In Sweden a law came into force in March 1985, giving an AID child the right of access to information on his genetic father when he or she reaches maturity. The counsellor can arrange for the donor and child to meet if both agree. This has bought about a decline in the numbers of couples requesting AID and there is some evidence that couples may be seeking AID abroad. There is also a change in the kind of men who become donors. They now tend to be married men with families rather than young, single men.

It is evident that strict checks on the kind of people who want to donate would be a good thing. At the moment, in London,

50 per cent of potential donors have to be excluded because they are carrying sexually transmitted diseases.

Offsetting such worrying statistics, other research shows that, in fact, donors tend to be very aware of what they are doing and have given responsible thought to it. The study of AID programmes in Melbourne by Robyn Rowland, quoted on page 70, interviewed 67 donors and found, surprisingly, that 42 per cent of them would still donate if their names were made available to the recipient couple. Most wanted to know if a child had been conceived with their sperm. Forty-eight per cent said that they would or did feel a connection with their offspring. A full 60 per cent said that they would not mind if their AID offspring contacted them after the age of 18, in order to discuss family background and so on.

Other donor's reactions to being contacted later in life are very different. In an article in *The Independent* newspaper on 6 July 1988, sperm donor 'Tom' is quoted as saying, 'I'd stop. It would put me at risk. People would find out. I would keep off registers at all cost.'

Dilemmas for the donor

The present situation where records do not exist is clearly unsatisfactory to the AID child who may one day discover a deep desire to trace his genetic father or whose life may even depend on this. If an AID child or adult needed a life-saving operation such as a bone marrow or kidney transplant, the donor or another of his offspring could save his life. In a case that arose in the USA in 1981, the courts refused to reveal a donor's name when someone conceived through AID needed a bone-marrow transplant. However, because of this possibility, the government of Victoria, Austrialia, passed legislation protecting the donor's anonymity while allowing him to be traced in such an emergency. AID centres must be approved by the health commission and information about the donor is passed on to the couple. Also, the donor may request some information on any children born as a result of his donation.

At the moment the exact status of the AID father were he to be identified is uncertain. Many donors may wish for anonymity to be protected only so that they will not find themselves liable to pay maintenance for the child at some later date. Most donors seem not to be averse to the idea of a national register where non-identifying information would be kept for the AID offspring at a later date. But since there is no clear policy on this, many British hospitals have destroyed all records and neither donors nor children have any hope of finding out about one another should they wish to do so.

The men questioned in the Melbourne study had given thought to many of the complex issues involved, although many of them wished there had been more opportunity to discuss the implications of donating sperm and of forming an opinion on many of the important issues. The sort of worries that could be aired are highlighted in this quote from a medical student who gave sperm:

'The first time I went, I felt for a moment I couldn't go through with it, it was such an eerie thing, thinking that I could be creating a child that I would never see. Now that I've got children of my own I do think about it sometimes. I've told my wife, but we've not told the children; they're too young to understand. Of course it's occurred to me, what if one of my daughters met a boy conceived with my sperm (who would be eight or nine years older). I don't know whether it would be such a good idea to put the idea into their heads. I'd be likely to see anyone they decided to marry, I suppose, and know if there were a strong resemblance ... it's so unlikely, it's not worth wasting time thinking about it really! (This possibility is further discussed below.)

Screening and other safeguards

Most doctors and clinics 'screen' donors – this may simply involve an interview to establish that there are no genetic diseases in the donor's family, that he is healthy and reasonably intelligent, and that he seems reasonably well-balanced.

The donors are often 'matched' with the husband – certainly for race, but also for other obvious characteristics such as hair colour, skin tone, eye colour, height and build. This is done to try to make the AID conception less obvious to an outsider, and spare the child from endless jokes about the milkman.

However, matching the donor and husband can also help the

couple to deceive themselves and convince themselves that perhaps the child really was the husband's after all. There is some degree of double-think going on here. Many couples are told to go home and make love after the wife has been inseminated so that they will never know for sure that the child is not their husband's. Some clinics mix the donor and husband's sperm for the same reason, though this practice tends to be frowned upon nowadays.

Other doctors may tell the couple to accept that the child is not the husband's and that he should come to terms with his infertility. Yet the donor is still chosen to look as much like him as possible. How would a couple react if the child did turn out to look very different from the 'father'? Would this affect how well the child is accepted by the family?

Donors are usually asked to limit the amount of sperm they give, to guard against the possibility of AID offspring marrying other children genetically related to them – in fact, their half-brothers and sisters. A limit of ten children per donor has been suggested by the Warnock report.

The fear of half-sibling marrying, however, is more of a psychological fear than a real possibility; it has been estimated in the USA that if one per cent of the population results from AID and each donor produces ten children, there would be less than one such marriage in 20 years. This is probably less than the number occurring because of children conceived through extra-marital affairs or from the adventures of a latter-day Don Juan. However, there is a case to be made for allowing children conceived through AID to check that if they marry another AID child, the donor is not the same.

Restricting donations to ten children may not be easy, though. Some clinics use donors many times, because they are reliable and suitable. And because it may take a woman many cycles of insemination to conceive, quite a lot of sperm may be needed.

In addition, many clinics want to keep more than one or two samples so that the couples have the choice of using the same donor for subsequent children. However, this may not always be possible. It takes an average of six months for most couples to conceive naturally and with AID this may be a little longer.

If they take some months to conceive on both occasions, it is unlikely that there would be enough sperm stored to enable the couple to choose the same donor. Indeed, often different donors are used at each visit, a fact which may cause concern to some women:

'When I asked was it the same donor, they said no, probably not. I thought that was very odd, having a different man's sperm every month. It made me feel a bit promiscuous.'

To some couples, the fact that their children should be full brothers or sisters seems very important, although there is no evidence to suggest that these children would get on any better than they would if they had different genetic fathers. The family environment seems more important in creating the feelings and emotions of brothers and sisters rather than the genetic link.

Relatives or friends as donors

Having a genetic link and knowing where your child came from is more important for some couples than others. As we saw in the section on surrogate mothers couples do not like the idea of an anonymous donor and have asked whether it would be possible if a male relative or friend could be used instead. Usually such suggestions are rejected by medical practitioners in Britain, although it is possible that some private doctors would arrange such a service. The NHS is unlikely to go along with such an arrangement, and the British Pregnancy Advisory Service, the largest provider of AID services outside the NHS, have a policy of only using anonymous donors. If doctors do not agree, couples may do it themselves at home, using 'self insemination techniques', or even ask for AIH and take the chosen donor's sperm in place of the husband's.

In the USA, doctors are more likely to go along with the couple's wishes, and known donors have certainly been used. One couple asked a brother, uncle and nephew of the husband, all single, to produce semen samples so the doctor could assess who would make the best donor. The doctor froze semen from all three and would not let the couple know whose sperm was eventually used, to try to prevent problems arising within the family. But arguably, many would feel it was better to know and, indeed, that this might even prevent family arguments.

Another couple did the insemination themselves with a friend's sperm in their own home. The wife said, 'I am very happy with our decision. I could never have carried a stranger's baby in my womb.' They report that three years later, the occasional visit of the genetic father and his wife creates no problems.

Caroline's story

Sometimes AID stories have fairy-tale happy endings. Caroline was a single woman who was refused AID when she decided she must have a baby before it was too late, but did not at that time have a relationship with a man. Friends said they knew someone who would make the ideal father; the couple met, discussed the situation and decided they felt very happy about the arrangement. The potential father would have no ties but would like to hear how his child got on. Caroline felt happy with the idea of this well-balanced, attractive man being the father of her child. 'I felt I would have good things to say about him if the child asked questions, as I knew he would, about the father.'

The couple first used self-insemination techniques but when this did not work the first two months, the decided to try the 'natural' way. A child was conceived and Caroline wrote informing the father about the progress of the pregnancy and birth. When the child was born, the father wrote and asked if she would mind him coming to see his son. His visits became very frequent, and in the end the couple fell in love and married.

Caroline felt that they had been mutually attracted at the first meeting. 'He was free, so was I, and we both liked the idea of having a child. If we had found one another repulsive, obviously we wouldn't have gone ahead. So I suppose the whole thing was set up from the beginning. How strange to live in a world where you can ask someone if you can bear their child at the first meeting, but not suggest you might get married.'

Superbabies

Some sperm banks in the USA have raised other problems by selecting Nobel-prizewinners as sperm donors, offering the sperm for use by women who want to produce a super-intelligent child.

In fact, there is no evidence that intelligence is passed on from parents to children in a simple fashion; intelligence tends to level out, and a high-achieving person is as likely to be motivated by aspects of his personality or by his family background and childhood experiences as by his intellect alone – none of which can be passed on. However, the idea of selecting donors for such qualities or indeed selecting recipients in a similar way is clearly disturbing, as is briefly discussed in Chapter 6.

5

Who's left
holding the baby?

Artificial reproduction is here to stay – but who will be able to take advantage of it? Although several thousand babies have now been born in Britain alone through IVF, there is still very little provision on the National Health Service (NHS) – at the time of writing. Most people can only get IVF privately, and at a cost that may put it out of their reach.

Similarly low prospects apply to those seeking Artificial Insemination by Donor (AID) treatment. Because so few NHS AID clinics exist the waiting lists are long; many patients have to wait one or two years before treatment. Consequently, private clinics in Britain are doing well.

Many people also have to wait up to 30 weeks between being referred by their GP and their first visit to the specialist. Even then, there may be long waiting times between tests and treatment. The one totally-NHS funded clinic at St Mary's Hospital, Manchester has a four year waiting list and cannot accept patients from outside the region. The Hammersmith Hospital in London has a two–three year waiting list.

Waiting lists present a particular problem to the infertile couple wherever they live, as many do not have much time. If a couple decide to start a family in their early 30s, as is more and more likely, it may be a year or two before they realise they have a problem. If they then see their doctor they may have to wait several months before they are referred to an infertility clinic or gynaecologist, by which time they will be about 35.

Infertility investigations may go on for up to a year, or longer, as many have to be carried out at certain times in the woman's menstrual cycle. Also, since ovulation may fall at a weekend or during holidays, it is not always possible to carry out tests in every cycle. Even when the problem has been identified there may be a further long wait for treatment, and the treatment may have to be carried out over a long period – with the possibility that it will have to be repeated several times.

Unfortunately, as the woman gets older her fertility declines and if she is eventually referred for IVF she simply may not have a year or two in which to wait. While about 90 per cent of women in their 20s will conceive within one year of regular sexual intercourse without contraceptives, only about 75 per cent of women will do so in their late 30s. Very few NHS clinics will treat an infertile woman once she reaches the age of 40, when the chances of treatment proving successful become very slim indeed, even if she can find a gynaecologist willing to help her. There are too many risks involved – for her and the baby.

Private medicine does not offer much help these days for the infertile either. The really well-off may attend private clinics, but even the private medical insurance companies are now trying to discharge this liability. While some used to pay for two or three attempts at IVF, they have now decided that infertility cannot be classified as an illness or injury and therefore is not eligible for cover. Another argument is that IVF does not 'cure' infertility but simply bypasses it – it does not restore the damaged tubes.

One of the major problems with commercial IVF clinics is that they are geared to IVF and do not necessarily offer other, less costly infertility treatment. There is, in fact, some evidence that patients are being given IVF treatment when their case could have been better met with microsurgery or with fertility drugs.

The fact that many people have to travel long distances to an area where infertility treatment is provided adds even more to the burden of cost. And as many infertility tests demand that you are close to the clinic, hotel expenses may also have to be taken into account.

Many infertile couples are so desperate for a child that they are prepared to pay dearly and to wait as long as necessary for infertility treatment. Others may decide to 'do it themselves'. Couples waiting up to two years for AID treatment when the man proves infertile might decide that a brief encounter with a discreet male friend might be the best solution. Infertile women unable to get IVF treatment may try to find a surrogate mother willing to have a baby for them.

SUITABILITY FOR TREATMENT

Infertile couples are not only prevented from receiving treatment in many cases because they live too far from a treatment centre of may not be able to afford expensive private treatment; other barriers exist too. Because demand far exceeds the availability of specialist help, doctors are frequently put in a position where they feel that only the most 'needy' can be offered treatment. Further, many doctors want to take couples for whom they feel there is a greater chance of success – because this is the best use of their resources, and because every doctor wants to achieve the highest possible success rate for his programme.

Many clinics therefore set criteria for who they will accept. They may specify that the couple have to be married or at least, living in a stable union. They may give preference to those who have no previous children – though some mothers are as desperate to have a second child as to have a first and some couples in second marriages want a child of their own as well as a stepchild. Many clinics will not take single women, lesbian women or women with a physical disability. Many will not treat women who are over 40.

In fact, all lesbian women have to do to achieve treatment, if they know it will not be offered to them if they admit their sexual orientation, is to keep quiet about it – if the clinic does offer treatment to single heterosexual women. However, the fact that they may have to lie to get treatment is not very helpful to anyone concerned.

While women in these situations feel that they should not be discriminated against because of their single status or sexual orientation, many health professionals feel that they have to consider the potential child – the kind of family he or she would be born into, and whether they would have a reasonable start in life. Many children are, in fact, being brought up in lesbian households, following divorce or a lesbian couple deciding to have a child with the help of a male friend, but society disapproves of such situations and the child is likely to experience hostility or prejudice from the outside world. Some doctors are reluctant to help create a child who may grow up with these problems.

Ethical considerations

Wherever there is a shortage of medical services seemingly arbitrary decisions about who should receive treatment are inevitably made. For example, if there are too few kidney machines doctors would tend to give priority to a young father of two rather than an elderly widower with no dependants. However, assessing the suitability of couples for infertility treatment can be rather more subjective. A couple turned down for IVF because they were 'too old' spoke out with great anger about these kinds of decisions:

'People do not ask if you are a young, married, morally upright character before giving you a heart transplant operation or some other major surgery which might save your life – and incidentally therefore enable you to become a parent later on,' said the woman. 'Yet they will turn you down for new infertility treatments because they consider you will not make a "suitable parent". We were turned down to adopt because of our age and because my husband once had a conviction for some minor incident years ago – when he was only in his teens. For the same pathetic reasons they are now denying us IVF.'

Doctors, with the best of intentions, are often trying to assess who would make the best parents – but this is something that cannot really be predicted in advance. In Britain, NHS IVF and infertility centres have ethical committees to help resolve such dilemmas. These committees have lay as well as medical people sitting on them, and are set up along guidelines provided by the Royal College of Physicians. However, some doctors are concerned at the role played by such committees and what their involvement should be. Ian Craft, who set up the IVF centre at the Royal Free Hospital and is now working at the Humana Hospital Wellington, feels that they are getting involved in clinical decisions which should be left to the doctor and his patient. 'A survey of infertile patients at the Wellington shows that they think that these committees should keep to purely ethical issues and not be concerned with clinical decisions.

'The trouble is that every individual is different, and I think it is wrong to have a distant body making decisions about an individual woman they don't know. It is no good saying, for instance, that a woman can only receive four eggs, if she needs more to get pregnant. People don't come to us to be partially treated, they come to have a child.'

As the number of embryos transferred is increased, the chance of a successful pregnancy increases, but so does the risk of a multiple birth. However, there is no way of predicting how such a transfer will result in any one woman. 'We transferred four embryos for one woman, and she had triplets – two of them identical. On the only occasion in which 12 embryos were transferred, in Germany, to a woman who had polycystic ovary disease, the result was one little girl.'

Ian Craft feels that some rulings also lead to difficult ethical problems. 'For example, if we collect and fertilise a number of eggs from a Catholic woman, she may insist they are all replaced because she cannot accept their destruction. In limiting the numbers of eggs that can be replaced, we may actually be preventing a woman having implanted into her womb her own eggs which have been fertilised by her partner. I think it is the woman who should make the choice of how many eggs should be implanted.'

The issue of selective reduction of multiple pregnancies is very complex. It has been strongly argued that the pregnancy is *not* actually being terminated, and the purpose of reduction is to maximise the chances of the outcome being successful. However, multiple pregnancies may come about by accident – through identical twinning of replaced embryos or over-stimulation of the ovaries with fertility drugs. If they do, the question arises whether it is better to let the multiple pregnancy continue with the additional risks to mother and babies, or whether to reduce the number of embryos to a safer and more acceptable level. The tragic case of the Halton septuplets highlights this problem (see page 52).

In such circumstances, many people believe, a selective reduction which would have enabled two or three healthy infants to have been born would have been preferable. As Ian Craft points out, 'No-one wants to undertake a selective reduction lightly. But, are you prepared to stand by and watch a pregnancy compromised and do nothing, when at the same time 170,000 abortions are being performed each year for purely social reasons?'

Mrs Aivazian, a patient of Ian Craft's, delivered a healthy baby girl on New Year's day on her 45th birthday, following a selective reduction from twins to a single foetus. She had been married for 14 years and lost seven pregnancies including one at 14, another at 23 and a third at 27 weeks. Because of her history of miscarriage, it was almost guaranteed that she would lose twins. 'No-one likes to do this, but I had to ask myself, would my conscience allow me to let her lose both those twins because I had scruples about carrying out a selective reduction?'

Assessing priorities when fertility treatment is short can indeed be very hard. One paediatrician I interviewed deplored multiple births resulting from fertility treatment and the medical care most needed. Many of these multiple births could have been avoided. 'I recall one occasion when six embryos were transferred to a woman, resulting in the birth of six premature, low-birth-weight babies. These clogged the neonatal unit of the Royal Free Hospital for a couple of months, meaning that other babies had to be turned away. I wonder how many parents who had just one baby today have no child because of this.'

Another issue about which there are strong feelings is egg donation by sisters. For many couples, this is the only possibility because there is such a shortage of anonymous egg donors. As we saw in Chapter 4, since the procedure involves an operation and an anaesthetic the main source of donated eggs is usually from friends or sisters of an infertile woman or from women on infertility programmes who produce an excess of eggs and want to donate them. Unfortunately, many women receiving fertility treatment – particularly older ones – may not make the best donors. The first pregnancy from a donated egg (mixed with donated sperm to make a 'donor embryo') in Australia, resulted in a miscarriage at ten weeks and the foetus was shown to have a chromosomal abnormalty. The egg donor was 42, an age at which the risk of conceiving a child with a chromosomal abnormality is comparatively high.

Even were anonymous donors more widely available, many women prefer to have their sister's eggs, so that the child will be more closely related to them. Some gynaecologists feel this decision is up to the couple entirely.

Another issue of concern is whether couples should be selected for their suitability to be parents before receiving infertility treatments. It has even been suggested that couples receiving IVF or other new fertility treatments should be assessed as are adopting couples.

In 1987, a woman revealed during counselling for IVF treatment at St Mary's Hospital, Manchester, England, that she had once worked as a prostitute. This was reported to the doctors who then decided not to proceed with IVF treatment, although for nearly a year the woman was not told of the real reason why she was refused treatment, despite seeing the doctors in the meantime. The case was discussed by the hospital ethical committee who confirmed the decision that she should not be given treatment. This rather disturbing case also raises the question of what is the difference between confidential counselling and vetting?

Importance of counselling

If information given in confidence to a counsellor is then reported to doctors who might decide against treatment, obviously patients will be reluctant to raise any doubts or emotional problems they might be feeling. Some couples will feel that if they admit, for example, that one of them had a temporary drink problem, had had a brief affair or had seen a psychotherapist as a result of depression related to the stress of infertility, they might be refused treatment, while concealing such potentially harmful facts would result in stress. This undermines the whole purpose and effectiveness of counselling, intended as it is to help the patient work out their own feelings and come to a decision as to what is best for them. Concealing fears and worries will not help couples overcome their difficulties or feel more positive about themselves before going ahead with treatment.

If infertile couples are to make considered decisions about what is best for them, counselling should help them to fully understand the implications of using donor sperm, eggs or embryos, to decide whether they would prefer known or unknown donors and to appreciate what their relationship would be with the child and with any third parties involved.

Many people believe that it is in any event wrong for anyone else to assess an infertile couple's suitability to have children, as no-one assesses the suitability of those couples lucky enough to be able to conceive naturally. However, assisted reproduction techniques where a donor or third party are involved do carry further implications, and a doctor may be reluctant to offer treatment using, say, donor sperm when he sees that the husband is clearly very unhappy about this.

This is why sensitive and enlightened counselling is so important. Following such counselling doubts and fears may be removed; or the couple may decide to drop out of the programme of their own accord. A small percentage of couples given counselling for AID do decide not to go ahead with the procedure, and some drop out after a few (unsuccessful) inseminations because they find the procedure too stressful or realise that they do not want to go through with it. As one woman explained:

'I hated AID ... the idea of someone else's sperm swimming inside me. I persevered for three months, and I didn't conceive, and when I was supposed to go back for the fourth time I felt sick at the thought. We talked it all over and I said, "It won't do, it's your child I want, not any old child. Let's forget it." John was delighted and said he had secretly dreaded it, too. He was going along with it for my sake. I'm glad that we got it out in the open because I'm sure it would have been a dreadful mistake and probably have destroyed our marriage, whereas now it is closer than it has ever been.'

Another problem that worries both counsellors and many

doctors is that when techniques are new and often experimental, some doctors will perhaps try out variations of that treatment not simply to see if this will improve the success rate but even just to 'see what happens'. Some of the results of such experimentation are bound to go wrong, just as others produce a 'miracle baby'. Yet how much should infertile women have to bear the consequences of new techniques which went wrong? Most patients are so desperate for a child that they are prepared to attempt anything, but is it ethically right to allow them to do so? And should they not at least be thoroughly counselled first?

Although infertility counselling is becoming more widely available, there is still a need for improvement. As infertility treatments become more complex and involve more and more ethical implications, it is vital that people considering such treatments should have a chance to think about and discuss the implications carefully with counsellors and medical staff.

Sometimes decisions made in a hurry might not have turned out for the best. Michelle and her husband, Joe, for example, were receiving test-tube baby treatment. Michelle had had fertility drugs and a laparoscopy for egg collection (see Chapter 4) and Joe was asked to produce a sperm sample (his sperm count had been tested before and was considered on the low side, but adequate). The sperm count on this occasion, however, was found to be too low for fertilisation to be successful.

'This put us under terrible pressure,' recalls Michelle. 'They said they could go ahead using donor sperm. We were all geared up to go so we said "yes" without really thinking it through. All the time we were waiting to hear if I was pregnant, I was terrified that on the one hand I might not be, and the effort would be wasted, and on the other that I was, and that it wouldn't be Joe's child. Fortunately, that time it didn't take. We then decided that Joe would provide some sperm that was OK and could be stored frozen so that we could fall back on that next time.'

Knowing in advance that such an option was available would have taken some of the pressure off. 'The stress is so enormous,' says Michelle, 'that it becomes hard to make the best decision. You don't know what is for the best. Because you want a baby so desperately you get carried away with that.

Then when you have time to think it through, you realise there might have been other choices. It wasn't quite so "now or never" as you saw it at the time.'

Good counselling is certainly likely to help protect the interests of the children who will be born as a result of these treatments, by enabling their parents to look into the future, see what problems they are likely to experience and helping them to come to terms with these possibilities so that they will not inflict their traumas on the child. Counselling is needed to help couples come to terms with their infertility, to understand the treatment they will receive, to explore their feelings towards bringing up a child which may not be genetically theirs and to think about how they will talk to the child about his or her origins when the time comes.

Counselling should certainly be seen as an essential part of any infertility service, anywhere in the world, and not just an 'optional extra'.

6

Embryo research – the vital issues

The new technology which has led to IVF, to the storage of frozen sperm, eggs and embryos, and their transference into the genetic mother or surrogate's body, has created new dilemmas. First of these is the question of who the sperm, eggs and embryos belong to:

- To the donor or genetic parent?
- To the recipient couple?
- To the doctors or hospital running the programme?
- To society at large?

Further, is the embryo a person or does it still have the status of egg and sperm separately? And whatever the answer to that one, who makes decisions concerning their future?

The storage of sperm, eggs and embryos has also made it possible for a baby to be conceived after one parent – or even both – have died. And that gives rise to many different problems, and reactions.

STORED SPERM

Men obliged to undergo medical treatment that might make them infertile – for example radio- or chemotherapy for

93

cancer, or surgery to remove the prostate gland – may have some of their sperm frozen so that they can start a baby later. In some cases, where the therapy has been unsuccessful and the man has died, the wife has still chosen to be inseminated with her husband's sperm.

This has already happened – probably many times – although if the sperm have been stored in a public hospital the health authority may not allow the frozen sperm to be released.

Many ethical and legal problems have been raised. For example, it has been pointed out that a man's estate could not be settled if there was a possibility that more children might be born to him in the future. Also, in Britain, the child could not be held to be legitimate under present legislation. The Warnock committee report made strong recommendations against the practice, because it also may give rise to profound psychological problems for the child and the mother.

Particularly complex is the case of David and Sonia Palmer. Before his death from cancer in 1985, David had banked sperm in the hope that he would recover and be able to have a child. After his death his wife applied to the hospital to have his baby. Sonia Palmer was already enrolled in the hospital's IVF programme because she had blocked Fallopian tubes.

Because Sonia's chance of conceiving was thought to be as low as one-in-six, her sister Carole then volunteered to act as surrogate mother. Both sisters were happy with this arrangement. Carole said, 'I know what I am taking on. I have to do this for Sonia. She wants David's child more than anything in the world and I can give it to her. She would do the same for me if the situation was reversed.'

Sonia, too, said: 'We are aware of the problems. We have talked this over for hours on end. It's not as if we are hiring a womb like other surrogates. It is being done for love, not money.' However, David's family were less than happy about the arrangement. His mother commented that this was 'turning her son into a circus'.

In August 1984 a French woman named Corinne Parpalaix was granted the right to be inseminated by her dead husband's sperm, which he had deposited at a sperm bank before receiving treatment for an illness that he was told would make him sterile. Corinne's request for the sperm was refused by the bank on the grounds that it had not been instructed by her husband to relinquish it to her. The judge ruled that sperm banks had no right to withold sperm in this way.

Corinne's brave attempt to have her late husband's child failed because the insemination treatment did not make her pregnant, but other French women now have the right to receive their dead husband's sperm. In the United States also, women have had babies after the husband's death, using banked sperm. The most well-known is Kim Cavali, creator of the popular 'Love is' cartoon, who had a baby a couple of years after her husband Roberto died of cancer.

STORED EGGS AND EMBRYOS

The same issues can arise where eggs or embryos are stored. It seems that sperm, eggs and embryos would be viable for at least ten years after storage. If a couple kept frozen sperm, eggs or embryos for future use, what would happen if either or both parents died, or if they divorced? Should a divorced woman be able to be implanted with an embryo conceived with her ex-husband's sperm?

If the genetic parents both agree, the embryo could be destroyed or donated, according to their wishes. But what if the couple disagree? Should the genetic parents make such decisions or should they be left to the hospitals, doctors and committees?

The Warnock committee in Britain recommended that storage of eggs, sperm and embryos by freezing should be permitted under licence. The donor's wishes should be carried out, and if the donor had died or could not be traced, the responsibility would pass to the Statutory Licensing Authority.

A government Bill intended to implement many of the proposals in the Warnock report provides that embryos should be stored for a maximum of five years and gametes for ten, with the signed consent of donors and for purposes only specified in that consent, for example, for treatment or research. Embryos should not be implanted, used for research or destroyed before the time limit expires without the consent of both donors. If a couple disagree, the embryos would be kept in storage till the time limit expired.

The idea that embryos stored by a couple for their own use and in the event not needed will be destroyed causes much anxiety in the minds of those who believe life begins at fertilisation. They criticise doctors for stimulating ovaries to produce more eggs than can be used at one time or fertilising more than can be implanted. In practice, it is hard to know whether eggs or embryos will be needed or not. It depends on how long it takes the woman to achieve a successful pregnancy (see Chapter 4).

One possibility is couples could donate unused eggs originally stored for their use. Isabel Bainbridge, who spent 17 years trying to overcome her infertility including five failed attempts at IVF, favoured this option. She could not understand why so much fuss was made about the loss of eggs or early embryos in IVF. 'In each ovary there are hundreds of eggs which die in various stages of development during a woman's lifetime. Every month nature causes eggs, embryos and sperm to die in a random fashion ... if I had my ovaries totally removed no-one would turn a hair, but because I have a couple of eggs removed, to be fertilised safe from the harm my body does to them, it turns many heads.'

While some couples undergoing IVF treatment are happy for their embryos to be donated to another infertile couple, others are not. As one woman said, 'It would be very disconcerting to know that somewhere there was another child of ours, a full brother or sister to our children. I don't think I could accept that very easily, unless we knew the couple and had contact. Even worse would be if their treatment succeeded and ours ultimately failed. It could all turn sour and cause pain. I think I would rather have any embryos left over destroyed or kept for our own personal use should we need it.'

STORAGE PROBLEMS

The freezing of sperm, embryos and eggs can be problematic in itself:

- About 50 per cent of sperm are killed in the freezing or thawing process, making it less successful in starting a pregnancy than fresh sperm. However, there is some evidence that more abnormal sperm are killed and thus the number of babies born with birth defects might be lower than in normal conception.
- When embryos are frozen, it is estimated that about 40 per cent will not survive the thawing process. This has led opponents of new reproductive technologies to describe embryo freezing as 'killing babies'.
- Egg freezing has so far been much harder to achieve, which is unfortunate since storing eggs and sperm separately might cause fewer ethical problems than storing embryos. There has been some concern that frozen eggs might result in embryos with more abnormalities than usual, though much more research in this area is needed. Despite such concerns, healthy babies have been born from frozen eggs. If the technology of egg freezing were improved, women could possibly store their eggs while young and use these eggs when they decide to have a baby later in life, thus avoiding the risks of a baby having Down's syndrome or other chromosomal abnormalities linked to increased maternal age.

EMBRYO RESEARCH

The most controversial area concerning the new reproductive techniques such as in vitro fertilisation is whether or not early human embryos should be used for research. The two sides in this ongoing debate have forceful arguments.

Those in favour, say that research on embryos could yield much information about human genetic disease, chromosomal disorders and other problems, possibly leading to their early detection or cure. They also argue that embryo research is vital in understanding why some early embryos implant and why so many others are lost. It might also help to improve the success of in vitro fertilisation programmes and help prevent miscarriages. Embryo research might also lead to new treatments for infertility, and to new and better methods of contraception. Almost all doctors and scientists in favour of embryo research believe that there should be strict controls on the research carried out, to prevent abuses, and that research should be restricted to a very early stage of embryonic development.

Those who are opposed to embryo research feel that this is the beginning of an unacceptable experimentation on human beings. They believe that human life begins with fertilisation and that no scientific goals can jusify such tampering with human life. They also fear that research on very early embryos will lead inevitably to later and later research on embryos.

HOW ABNORMALITIES ARISE

Before addressing the question of whether research on early human embryos can be justified, it helps to understand how abnormalities arise. The causes can be either environmental – such as poor diet in the mother, the use of certain drugs in early pregnancy or exposure to toxic chemicals or radiation – or genetic. Genetic problems fall into two categories: those caused by either or both parents carrying a faulty gene, or those which occur when the egg and sperm are formed or fuse and involve an extra chromosome or part of a chromosome being included in the fertilised egg.

Chromosomes are the essential components of every living cell, determining not only how each cell works, but how the whole organism develops, functions and looks. The chromosomes are made up of smaller units called genes, each of which determines a particular characteristic of the organism. Every animal and plant species has its unique number and size of chromosomes – in humans there are 46 chromosomes in 23 pairs. In each individual, one set is inherited from the mother and one set from the father.

When the human cells divide to create the sperm and the egg, the pairs of chromosomes mix and separate at random so that each egg and sperm carries a different set of genes on the

23 chromosomes, although there will always be one of each pair (unless something has gone badly wrong). This is why every human being is different. One of the pairs of chromosomes determines the baby's sex; these are called the X and Y chromosomes, because of their shape when viewed under the microscope. When sperm are formed, half will carry the X and half the Y chromosome, while all eggs carry the X chromosome.

Very occasionally the process of division will go wrong and the sperm or egg cell will end up with an extra chromosome or part of a chromosome. In such instances, when sperm and egg fuse the embryo will be faulty. Most faulty embryos cannot survive for long, and it is thought that as many as 50 per cent of recognised spontaneous abortions or miscarriages are caused by the embryo being abnormal. Many more early miscarriages are perhaps never even recognised.

Sometimes the presence of an extra chromosome does *not* prevent the baby from developing or living. The most common problem of this nature is when there is an extra one of the 21st pair of chromosomes, which causes Down's syndrome. Other chromosomal abnormalities which are not lethal are when a girl lacks an X chromosome (Turner's syndrome) or a boy has an extra X or extra Y chromosome. Turner's syndrome results in a girl who is of small stature and will be sterile. An extra X chromosome in men causes Klinefelter's syndrome, which results in them having a slightly feminine physique and being infertile.

Other genetic diseases and handicaps are caused by a faulty gene. Literally hundreds of inherited diseases or syndromes are now known, although most are extremely rare. Some are caused by a dominant gene and others, more commonly, by a recessive gene.

A dominant gene will always show itself when present, while a recessive gene can remain hidden, perhaps for generations, till it pairs up with another recessive gene for the same condition. Two relatively well-known dominantly inherited diseases are Huntington's chorea, a degenerative nerve disease which does not show up till the third or fourth decade of life, and achondroplasia, a form of dwarfism which occurs more often when the father is older. If a person has a dominantly inherited disease, the chance of their child being affected is 50 per cent.

Recessively inherited diseases can be carried by large numbers of people without their knowledge. As long as the recessive gene is paired only with normal genes, there is no problem. However, if both partners carry the abnormal gene, there is a one-in-four chance of their children having the disease; and a fifty per cent chance that their children will be carriers.

Recessively inherited diseases include cystic fibrosis, Tay Sachs disease, sickle-cell anaemia, and phenylketonuria. Some of these can be treated if diagnosed early, such as phenylketonuria, by putting the child on a special diet. Others can be tested for during pregnancy, although this may induce a miscarriage.

If an abnormal gene is carried on one of the sex chromosomes, the disease is said to be sex-linked. The female X chromosome is longer than the male Y chromosome and carries many more genes. If one of these is abnormal, it will usually be masked by a normal corresponding gene on the X chromosome pair. If paired with a Y chromosome, however, the condition will show itself. So, sex-linked diseases are much more common in boys. Examples of sex-linked diseases are Duchenne muscular dystrophy and haemophilia.

Some congenital abnormalities and diseases are caused by a combination of several faulty genes. There can be environmental factors too, such as the combination of a faulty gene with some other effect such as a drug taken in pregnancy or a faulty diet. It seems that neural tube defects (spina bifida and anencephaly), cleft palate and hair lip, and congenital heart abnormalities are caused in this way. There may also be a random element in some defects – there have been recorded cases of identical twins where one had a cleft lip and the other did not.

PREVENTING ABNORMALITIES

Understanding the mechanisms which lead to congenital abnormalities and genetic diseases is necessary before progress can be made in preventing or curing them.

Professor Robert Edwards, who developed the IVF technique in Britain with the surgeon Patrick Steptoe, points out that IVF would have been impossible without previous research on embryos. 'We had to do research before replacing an embryo in the mother, to ensure that the embryo was developing normally and that the chromosomes were right.

'Chromosomal abnormalities can arise in the embryo as it divides. One cell goes wrong, then continues to multiply. It is now thought that most Down's syndrome babies who survive till birth are "mosaics" – with a mixture of normal cells with 46 chromosomes and abnormal cells with 47. This may explain why some Down's syndrome babies are more severely affected than others. The defect must have arisen at an early division of the embryo, so understanding how this arises could be important in finding ways to prevent it.'

Chromosomal abnormalities are now a major cause of death of newborn babies, as deaths from other causes have steadily gone down thanks to better medical care. The prevention of such abnormalities is clearly very important in improving the mortality rate of newborns still further, and preventing the suffering of both child and family when a severely handicapped child survives.

The present 'prevention' of such tragedies comes about through detection of an abnormality fairly late in pregnancy, by a process known as an amniocentesis. In this test, amniotic fluid is drawn out of the mother's abdomen by a syringe and the foetal cells are cultured in a laboratory and then analysed. This is carried out at around 16-18 weeks of pregnancy and results take another two to three weeks.

Clearly, detection at a much earlier stage would lessen the trauma of having a late termination of pregnancy. Figures from the United States' National Institutes for Child Health show that 95 per cent of parents who discover their baby is abnormal decide on a termination. This is one of the most difficult decisions a couple can ever have to make, as by then the woman will have felt her baby moving and will be having a termination almost at the point when her baby could have survived had it been born prematurely.

A more recent technique known as Chorionic Villi Sampling

may ultimately replace amniocentesis as a method of diag-
nosing abnormalities. This test involves taking a sample of
tissue from the placenta with an instrument passed through the
cervix. It can be carried out as early as 8 weeks and gives the
mother the option of a quick, early abortion if her baby should
be found to be abnormal. However, at present the test carries
a higher risk of inducing a miscarriage – about one in 50 as
contrasted with one in 150 for amniocentesis. It may be that
this ratio will improve as people become more skilled in
performing Chorionic Villi Sampling, or it may be that passing
an instrument through the cervix inevitably carries more risk
of disrupting a pregnancy.

Bernadette Modell, Senior Lecturer in Perinatal Medicine
at University College Hospital, London, pointed out the
terrible toll that carrying genetic diseases can have on the
families. 'Though 25 per cent of the pregnant women at risk
of having thalassaemic infants who came to us had late
abortions ... a surprising number became pregnant again
very soon. Two unfortunate women each had five antenatal
diagnoses, and each had four pregnancies terminated at twenty
weeks because of a positive diagnosis.'

If abnormal embryos could be detected right at the beginning of their lives, a woman would never have to become
pregnant and then discover her baby was abnormal. If eggs are
fertilised outside the womb, they can be checked for
abnormalities before being transferred to the mother's womb.
This could be done for women who are at very high risk of
having an abnormal baby either because of their age or because
they carry a genetic disease.

Another possibility, for those who conceive naturally, is that
the embryos could be flushed out of the womb by the technique
called lavage, if this could be made safer than it is at present.
The embryo could then be checked and reintroduced.

One way of checking the embryo is by doing a 'biopsy' and
removing a cell from the growing embryo (which will continue
to develop normally) at an early stage when the embryo is just
a cluster of identical cells, all of which have the potential to
develop into any part of the body. A 'DNA gene probe' can be
used to latch on to and identify an abnormal gene within the
cell. This can be done for diseases such as cystic fibrosis,

thalassaemia, haemophilia, and some muscular dystrophies and will soon be extended to many other hereditary diseases. The embryo can also be checked for problems such as Down's syndrome, and abnormalities where the child has an extra sex chromosome as in Klinefelter's syndrome in boys with an extra Y chromosome, or has lost one as in Turner's syndrome in girls missing an X chromosome.

SCREENING FOR A PERFECT BABY?

One misgiving about genetic screening is that it will become possible for less and less handicapping conditions, such as cleft palate or some hereditary diseases which are not life-threatening. Embryos could also be 'sexed', allowing parents the choice of a boy or girl.

Even where an inherited disease is detected, such screening could not necessarily reveal the extent of the problem; many of the conditions vary in severity for reasons which are not fully understood. Is it right to stop an embryo from developing further on the basis of an uncertain diagnosis? Should the search for a 'perfect baby' be allowed to go this far?

Another possibility is that eggs could be split to create identical twins, one being watched in vitro while the other is replaced in the mother. She could then have her pregnancy terminated if the in vitro baby developed abnormally or had a genetic disease. However, the idea of creating such twins makes many uneasy, as it carries the possibility of creating identical individuals who could be implanted into a woman at different times, even skipping a whole generation.

WHEN SHOULD EMBRYO RESEARCH CEASE?

The second major issue is: up to what stage should research on embryos be allowed? Obviously there has to come a point where the embryo is considered sufficiently developed to make embryo research abhorrent to the great majority of doctors, scientists and laymen. That point is probably reached when the embryo has achieved a human form or could be capable of feeling pain. One suggestion is that research might be allowed up to 14 days from fertilisation, as this does provide a clear step on the slow path of the embryo from fertilised egg to fully developed foetus.

After the human egg has been fertilised the first divisions take place very slowly. Fertilisation itself is not a clear-cut process – once the sperm enters the egg the outer membrane of the egg becomes impermeable to further sperm, but it takes up to 24 hours for the chromosomes of the sperm to fuse with those of the egg. The first division then takes place, to be followed 12-24 hours later with a further division, and within a further 14-20 hours by another division to create an eight-cell embryo. At the fifth division, about five days after fertilisation, the embryo develops an inner layer and an outer mass and is called a blastocyst. The outer layer is needed to implant in the womb and forms the placenta, while the inner mass develops into the embryo proper.

The blastocyst continues to divide, more rapidly now, and by day six or seven begins to implant into the lining of the womb. Implantation takes about a week, and is usually completed by 12 – 14 days after fertilisation. The inner cell mass forms the embryonic disc and the forerunner of the spinal cord, known as the 'primitive streak', then emerges – the first clearly defined feature of the embryo. (Two primitive streaks can arise in the embryo, leading to the development of identical twins.)

The primitive streak is formed 14 – 16 days after fertilisation and many scientists argue that its emergence is the stage at which the embryo can be said to have become a biological individual. From then on development is rapid.

- At 17 days the first signs of the nervous system appear with the beginning of the spinal cord.
- By the end of the first month the beginnings of all the major organs can be seen and the cardiovascular circulation has begun.

- In the sixth week the arm and leg buds are formed and the brain and sex organs also begin to form.
- In the seventh week the beginnings of the fingers and toes are visible and dramatic changes are occurring to the head and face.
- In the ninth week the nose and mouth take shape.
- By the eleventh week the genital organs are formed and all the internal organs are functioning.
- The higher parts of the brain start to show electrical activity after about 12 weeks, when the foetus is fully formed.

From then on the foetus grows in size and matures, but the work of formation is basically completed. The 14-day limit does therefore have some logic about it and has received fairly widespread support. Many scientists argue that it is best to call the embryo up till 14 days a 'pre-embryo', as this helps make it clear in the public mind that what is being discussed is a group of cells with no human features; the term 'embryo' tends to conjure up the image of a miniature human with arms, legs, and a head.

Some scientists, like test-tube baby pioneer, Professor Robert Edwards, are against *any* arbitrary limit to research. 'I think this limit is nonsense; completely and utterly wrong. At present researchers have the right to use tissue from aborted foetuses up to, I think, six months. This is used widely to make vaccines. Corneas from foetuses are used for grafting, and trials are being carried out using nerve and brain cells from embryos for the treatment of Alzheimer's disease. This is already going on. Society cannot attack us for researching on a blastocyst when they are prepared to abort a healthy foetus at up to 24 weeks or more.'

At a study group that met at the Ciba Foundation, London, in November 1985 to discuss embryo research, Professor Edwards made clear his objection to a 14-day rule. 'I believe a better alternative to the 14-day rule is to establish a powerful ethical authority which demands justification for every piece of research. The 14-day rule is too generous for some research; for example, the study of chromosomes can largely (but not entirely) be done at day five. Studies on the differentiation of the haemopoietic (blood formation) system would require embryos at day 14 or perhaps later. For the myocardium (heart tissue) it would be necessary to go to day twenty. Each of these is a legitimate study, yet if an arbitrary line is drawn some of them are excluded.'

Many scientists however, are not reassured by the idea of an ethical body making such decisions. They feel that a line is necessary to reassure the public that embryo research is not going 'too far'. In so far as a line can be drawn, 14 days seems the most clearly defined and the most likely to be selected. In one sense such discussion is currently academic. The longest period during which embryos have been grown in vitro is nine days, at which point they had probably reached about the stage of a seven or eight-day embryo. One nine-day embryo attached to the plastic vessel and formed tissues. It seems important to set the boundaries of acceptable research before scientists exceed this. But allowing research even up to this point is not certain, and there are still more complex ethical questions to be examined.

FURTHER QUESTIONS

One question which has occupied those involved with embryo research is the origin of the embryos which are being used. Scientists have made a distinction between 'spare' embryos which were obtained originally for implanting into an infertile woman's womb but which were not then needed (perhaps because many healthy embryos were obtained, or because they were stored for later use and were not needed because the initial treatment was successful) and embryos created especially for research, perhaps from donated eggs and sperm. Some people feel happier about the use of 'spare' embryos, which exist and would have to be destroyed anyway, than about those created especially for research.

Another question is: what should be done with embryos which are considered not to be developing well enough to be put back into the mother, or which are abnormal. At the Ciba study group, Professor Edwards said that they used abnormal embryos for research, such as those with an extra set of 23 chromosomes (these embryos are known as triploid and will all spontaneously abort). 'This is very similar to the use of aborted material for research in other areas, such as making vaccines.'

Professor Edwards has held back from creating large numbers of embryos specifically for research. However, the technology is there and there is some concern that commercial laboratories may even be doing this for purposes which many would consider inappropriate – hence the need for careful regulation. There is a possibility that otherwise embryos could be grown by commercial companies to test out the toxicology of their products or to grow human 'spare parts' for transplants.

Yet there is also the possibility that some adult disease could be cured by using embryonic cells. For example, embryo stem cells, which are found in the part of the early embryo that later develops into certain organs, could replace bone marrow transplants for leukaemia patients. In the words of Professor Edwards, 'We could replace bone marrow which has been damaged by chemotherapy or radiotherapy with embryo stem cells, and make radiated, anaemic, damaged people normal. We wouldn't need bone marrow registries, we wouldn't need to match tissue and risk rejection.'

A team in Lyons, France recently reported that they had transplanted cells from aborted foetuses into 12 children with severe auto-immune deficiency disease who had previously had to live in isolation 'bubbles'. The transplanted stem cells were accepted by the infants and grew into normal white blood cells. It is also hoped that transplanting cells from the pancreas of foetuses might produce insulin-making cells in an adult diabetic, thus curing this disease.

There is a difference however between using foetuses which have already been aborted or, some argue, 'spare' embryos which have already been created and would otherwise be destroyed and using those created without any intention that they should develop into a person. Yet there are also many scientists who do not accept that there is a difference in using spare normal embryos or those created for research. They argue that either experimentation on early embryos is justifiable or it is not, regardless of the origin of the embryo.

Either the embryo must be protected as potential human life or not.

Of course, the fate of such an early embryo is uncertain. No-one can know whether it would develop into a viable human foetus or not. Many early embryos fail to implant. Why is not known, but it may be that there is a defect which prevents implantation. Many develop a placenta and other tissues but contain no embryo proper. These always result in miscarriages, and may be referred to as a 'blighted ovum'.

Some embryos may, rarely, develop into a hyatidiform mole – a collection of large undifferentiated cells which also results in a miscarriage and can be damaging to the mother if the tissues invade the walls of the womb – or even a teratocarcinoma, in which the embryo turns into an invasive growth. It is also very likely that, for a number of reasons, an embryo would be miscarried.

The fact that not all fertilised eggs are capable of developing into viable embryos does not, however, mean that they should not be treated with respect. Most people feel this strongly. Once a woman knows she is pregnant she usually looks forward to the birth of another human being even if it turns out that her pregnancy was not a good one from the outset and she miscarries a severely abnormal embryo, and will grieve that loss accordingly.

CLONING

Much of the opposition to embryo research comes from fears that, once allowed, research on embryos could lead to experiments such as 'cloning', a science-fiction process in which identical individuals could be produced from one embryo. In fact, cloning might be possible without using embryos at all. One human cell is all that would be necessary were the technique possible, as imagined in the film, *The Boys from Brazil*, in which clones of Adolf Hitler were adopted by carefully selected families as close to his own background as possible.

A limited form of cloning in the sense of producing genetically identical individuals is possible now. As we saw earlier in this chapter, if at the two-cell stage of development of an embryo fertilised in vitro the cells were separated, they could then develop into two genetically identical individuals. However, this is not likely to be very popular even if available. Most parents find one of the greatest pleasures of having more than one child is the difference in their looks and personalities.

Would it be possible to go on dividing the embryo and produce dozens of identical babies? In theory, this might be possible. And these identical embryos could be implanted into dozens of surrogate mothers, so that dozens of identical children were born. So, in a sense, cloning is possible already.

Clones can be produced from certain animals in the laboratory by a different technique. With frogs, toads and salamanders scientists can take the nucleus (containing the genetic material) from an embryonic cell and place it in an egg which has had its nucleus removed. The egg then develops as if it had been fertilised. Many eggs can be treated in this way with nucleii from the same embryonic tissue. However, doing this with mammalian cells is much more difficult. One scientist claimed success using this technique on mice, but the experiment has not been repeated.

The worse visions of cloning involve taking cells from a living adult – perhaps a mad dictator – or even a dead one – and creating identical individuals to perpetuate them for ever. Others involve developing a kind of superman through selective breeding and then thousands more in his image, perhaps to form an army.

Neither of these possibilities is remotely near, as there is no way at present of taking an adult cell and making it revert to the embryonic state where it is capable of developing into a whole individual. At a certain stage of development, cells lose their totipotency – their ability to develop into any kind of cell found in the human body.

GENETIC ENGINEERING

Another fear, linked to cloning, is the development of types of human beings through genetic engineering, perhaps the super-intelligent or the super-strong. Genetic engineering is a loose term which covers a range of processes where scientists might alter the genetic material in a cell. Genetic engineering might make possible the elimination of undesirable characteristics or the substitution of desirable ones. It might make possible the elimination of certain diseases and handicaps.

Another possibility which has raised alarm is that of trans-species fertilisation; that is, the fertilising of another animal's egg with human sperm, and vice versa. Doctors have fertilised hamster eggs with human sperm to see whether the sperm are capable of penetrating an egg and fertilising it. Any resulting embryo cannot develop beyond the two-cell stage. But supposing the embryo of a human and another animal were able to develop into a half-human, half-animal hybrid? It is thought that there is no animal close enough to humans genetically for this to be possible, but obviously it is an alarming prospect. Should further research in this area be banned?

The problem with all these issues is that, once they are technically possible, it is conceivable that an unscrupulous society might use them for the wrong ends. Of course, almost all scientific developments have the power to be used for good or for evil, but society must accept that the sorts of issues raised in this chapter are major ones and seek to regulate any practices which have a potential for misuse.

BEYOND THE WOMB

Another future possibility is that it may be possible for a foetus to develop outside the mother's womb, in a suitably contrived and controlled environment. This technique is known as ectogenesis. It is already possible for an embryo to be conceived and to spend its first days 'in vitro', outside the mother's womb, and to spend the last part of the pregnancy in an incubator. Babies born prematurely are now surviving routinely at 28 weeks gestation and some have been saved from as early as 21 or 22 weeks in exceptional circumstances.

However, such babies need feeding through a tube, their lungs must be ventilated and their tiny bodies kept warm. They may also need drugs and other treatments to fight off infections. These babies are denied the comforting sounds and motion of the mother's body and – who knows – may be denied other important elements of life in the womb.

Is it possible or desirable for a baby to be nurtured entirely in an artificial environment until it is ready to be 'born'? Some people argue that there is no reason why the age at which a baby can survive if born prematurely should not be pushed back to the beginning of its life. This would allow women who did not want their baby a choice not to have the pregnancy terminated but instead to surrender the embryo at a very early stage so that it could then be maintained till old enough to be given to adoptive parents. This might mean the end to abortion as we know it. And women unable to carry a baby in their womb would not have to resort to using a surrogate with the potential pitfalls involved (see Chapter 4). Doctors would be able to observe the development of the embryo and any handicaps could be spotted at an early stage.

However, some people fear that perhaps all women would then seek to be freed from the 'burden' of pregnancy. Nurturing a baby outside the womb, or ectogenesis as it has been termed, could become a matter for convenience. What effect would that have on the baby – or, indeed, on the mother?

Pregnancy is not necessary for mother-child bonding, as adoption and surrogate motherhood have clearly proved. However, the experience of being carried in the mother's womb may be a very important one for the baby. Research has shown that a newborn baby has learned to recognise the sound of the mother's voice from inside the womb – or at least to recognise the human voice.

EFFECTS OF PREMATURE BIRTH

Without a doubt, being born premature is traumatic for the baby, and its mother. Mothers whose very small babies have been maintained in an incubator for some time speak of their suffering as they watch and wait, helplessly. 'It was terrible to watch the doctors putting the feeding tube down her throat . . . she would go into convulsions of pain and fear,' said one mother. 'Because she was so covered with monitors and tubes and things it was impossible to hold her and comfort her properly. They found that by putting her on a soft surface instead of the flat hard sheets she did better . . . I am sure that a baby suffers from not being close to the mother, apart from all the painful procedures that have to be endured.'

Little research has been done to see what effects being born prematurely has on a child's psychological development. Nor has much been done to investigate the effect of birth. While many claims have been made regarding the effect of the birth trauma on people's personality, no research has looked at babies born by Caesarian who do not experience the normal birth process. However, the prospect of ectogenesis causes unease for most people and, if research is banned on embryos of more than 14 days gestation, the path to ectogenesis is likely to come from a gradual pushing back of the number of weeks at which premature babies can survive.

A MALE PREGNANCY?

In theory, a baby does not have to grow inside the womb; it can grow anywhere inside the mother's body. Ectopic pregnancies – which start outside the womb – usually occur within the Fallopian tube where the foetus cannot grow beyond a certain size without rupturing the tube, a potentially fatal event for the mother. However, pregnancies have established themselves elsewhere in the mother's abdominal cavity, although such a pregnancy would be very fragile as the foetus is not protected by the muscular womb. (There have been very rare instances of babies being born following an abdominal pregnancy, but the vast majority are lost.)

Recent speculation has included the possibility that a man could carry a baby in the same way, were he given suitable hormones to enable his body to support a pregnancy. Hormone treatment has been given to women without functioning ovaries to enable them to support a pregnancy. Hormones are needed for the first 50 days of the pregnancy, after which the developing embryo produces all the hormones needed and the pregnancy becomes self-sufficient.

Some scientists believe that hormone treatment might not even be necessary. In the 1960s, a male baboon was given a fertilised egg and carried it until it was deliberately aborted at four months gestation. It had been implanted in the abdominal wall, and attached itself to the fatty tissue which protects the large intestine. Other scientists believe that it would not only be necessary to give hormone treatments, but also to implant some tissue from the womb lining (endometrial tissue) with the embryo to help it to implant.

An embryo could be implanted into a man and attached to a suitable organ such as the kidney or wall of the large intestine, and continue to develop until it was ready to be born by a kind of Caesarian section. This operation could be dangerous to both father and baby, as great care would be needed to prevent a severe haemorrhage from the organ to which the placenta was attached.

Male pregnancy is an exciting idea to many people – as it would enable a couple to share the experience of parenthood totally and create more equality between the sexes. It would enable a husband whose wife cannot bear a child to do so in her stead, so avoiding the involvement of surrogates or outside parties. It would also enable homosexual couples to have 'their own' child (an egg would have to be donated). Yet the idea that men could become pregnant is abhorrent to others. And would the side-effects of a male pregnancy – treatment with female hormones, the risks to the man and baby – outweigh any possible advantages? At the moment, the answer is 'No'.

In all such possibilities, how the future child will feel about his origins and any suffering he has to undergo as a result of his unusual birth will have to be considered, just as it is in the case of other infertility treatments. In the next, and final, chapter we will consider how children who already live in unconventional families feel about their lives, to gain some insight into their likely feelings and concerns. This may also help couples considering new fertility treatments to anticipate and deal with any problems their children may have as a result of their own desire to have a child by any means.

7

Happy families – or strained relations?

How much can we predict about the feelings and problems likely to be faced by the children born of the new reproductive techniques? Because most are so new, there is little actual evidence available. However, there is a wealth of information that comes from existing families where the children are not the blood relatives of both parents – adoptive families and step-families. Although these families are in some respects very different, there are similar complexities in the relationships thus formed.

Those who have had or want to have children not genetically their own, whether through egg, sperm or embryo donation or through a surrogate mother – make it clear that the child will not suffer because it is wanted. However, most adopted children are also wanted and this does not seem to prevent some fundamental doubts and problems arising about their sense of worth and their identity. Many adopted children speak of the importance of having a sense of your own identity, of knowing where you belong and how you came there. Do children have this right, and if not, how are they going to feel about it?

In Chapter 4, we have already learned a little about such issues; this chapter will examine in depth the kinds of situations and emotions with which the children, parents and other relatives will be faced as a result of the new reproductive technologies, and what sort of resolutions they may come to.

115

Each situation is likely to be unique, because each family will be unique, but many of the underlying doubts and tensions may be the same. In any event, these problems are not going to go away because we ignore them, and those who are considering embarking on a treatment which will result in a child conceived not wholly by them should certainly consider their feelings, their partner's feelings and those of the child before committing themselves to a final decision.

WHOSE CHILD AM I?

The importance of knowing one's identity has been acknowledged since ancient times, as expressed in myths such as that of Oedipus. When Oedipus was born it was prophesied that he would one day marry his mother and kill his father. He was abandoned on a mountainside to avoid this fate, but was found and raised by a peasant family in ignorance of his origins. So it happened that, when grown to manhood, he killed a stranger who turned out to be his father, and unwittingly married the woman who happened to be his mother. The words Sophocles puts into the mouth of Oedipus, 'I must pursue this trail to the end, till I have unravelled the mystery of my birth,' may find an echo among many adopted children and, indeed, children born of the new birth technologies.

Although the Oedipus story was intended to illustrate how we cannot avoid our fate, it also shows many of the fears we carry about not knowing who our parents are and why the fear of incest looms large in discussions of artificial insemination by donor and anonymous egg or embryo donation.

Many myths and fairy tales tell of the tragic consequences that befall people who are deprived of the knowledge of their origins. Others, however, end happily when the prince brought up by the peasant comes into his rightful heritage and marries the fairy princess. Even so, his correct identity and the story of his life have to be revealed before he can come into his kingdom.

Many legends and folk stories also tell of illegitimate children and the trouble they cause. Arthur's downfall came from his incestuous liaison with his aunt, Queen Morgan la Fay, and the resulting birth of Mordred, whose bitterness at not being acknowledged as his son and jealousy of those held in higher esteem caused him to reveal Lancelot's affair with Guinevere and precipitate the final conflict. Guinevere, incidentally, remained childless, and the fact that Arthur had no legitimate heir was a factor in bringing about the final tragedy.

Although many of the complexities in relationships made possible by assisted reproduction techniques may seem new, it is not difficult to find equivalents for those, too, in the past.

- The position of the AID child is similar to that of the child conceived by an unknown man with whom his mother had a brief relationship. Usually she will know who the man is and, rarely, may even tell the child about it or reveal the father's identity.
- The AID child might also be compared with the child whose stepfather brought him up from a very early age and who does not know his original father.
- The position of the child born from a donated embryo is similar to that of an adopted child.
- A child born from his maternal aunt's donated egg might be in a similar situation to a child who's mother gave him to her sister to bring up because the latter was infertile.

All these situations have existed for centuries. The only problem in using them as guides to what the future may hold for children born of the new techniques is that there has been no formal study of how children fare in most of these situations. Most of what we do know of how children feel about unorthodox beginnings has been gathered from studies of adoption.

All the major studies which have been carried out show that, in terms of overall development and achievement, adopted children do at least as well as other children. They also do better than children brought up in care and, as Barbara Tizard showed in her study, *Adoption: A Second Chance*, children may do better when adopted rather than reunited with their original families.

LATER EMOTIONAL PROBLEMS

There has been some debate about whether adopted children face a greater risk of developing emotional problems later in life. Some studies claim that adopted children show greater emotional vulnerability, and a higher incidence of personality disorders. However, the child's experience *before* being adopted is very important here. A child adopted at birth might be expected to have fewer problems than one adopted after an unhappy start in life.

Those who believe that adopted children might face problems connected with their origins, put forward several likely reasons:

- The first is to do with the parents' unresolved feelings and emotions about infertility, and the fertile partner's anger at the infertile one. The infertile partner might also have feelings of guilt or inadequacy, and the child might sense these unexpressed feelings.
- Secondly, the adoptive parent might be more anxious than usual, having become a parent only after many difficulties and feeling that they must excel in order to make up for the child's original loss. This may be made worse by having to go through rigorous screening to assess their 'suitability' to become parents. The child may also be seen as having to be 'special', to make up for not being their own.
- Children might fear that the original parents must be 'bad' to have abandoned them, or indeed that they must have been to blame for their parents' rejection of them. Researchers Simon and Sentura have written that they believe this original loss might lead to a depressive core, and a fantasy of reunion with the original parents to overcome this. A child might fear being abandoned again in the future and feel his or her good behaviour is necessary to prevent this.
- Above all, having two sets of parents – even if one set are

never known to the child – might cause difficulties for a young child's psychological development. The myth of the wicked stepmother comes out of the normal developmental process of splitting the good and bad aspects of a mother into two separate beings. The young child cannot accept that the mother could hurt him or deny him basic needs, so he projects hostile acts towards him onto another, 'bad' mother. Eventually he will be able to accept that the 'good' and 'bad' mothers are the same and fuse them into a whole. If, in fact, he does have another mother, be she birth mother, surrogate mother or stepmother, this process of fusion may be confused or delayed.

- In adolescence, a teenager aware of the fact that she is the child of someone other than the parents who brought her up might act more rebelliously or outrageously than the average teenager, out of a need to test her parents affection and also perhaps to show that she is different from them. This situation can be painful and confusing for all family members, and if handled badly, can result in more lasting problems.

FAMILY ROMANCE

A universal fantasy which is also relevant to this rationalising of children's behaviour, is that which Freud called the 'family romance'. In it, the child doubts that he is the natural child of his parents and fantasises about another set of parents who are usually more wealthy or powerful.

This fantasy is useful when the child feels angry or frustrated that the parents don't understand him or give him enough love. Once the child accepts that he can both love and hate the same person this fantasy is usually resolved. It may be more difficult for a child to use this fantasy if he or she realises that they had other parents about whom they know little.

In addition, if the 'other parents' are seen not to be higher in status but, in fact, lower, unmarried or very poor, this may make it hard for the child to hold the same images and fantasies as other children.

SPECIALLY CHOSEN

Many – perhaps the majority – of children who know they are adopted were told that they were 'specially chosen', to compensate for any possible feelings of rejection at being given up by their natural mother.

However, adopted children often feel they have to live up to their parents' high expectations, and must be perfect, or become what their parents want them to be and not themselves. The story, like denying adoption, is also based on falsehood, because most adopted children were not 'chosen' in this way. As an adoptee quoted in the American study *The Adoption Triangle* by Arthur D. Sorosky, Annette Baran and Reuben Pannor, remarks of this myth, 'As if my adoptive parents picked me from a cast of thousands rather than gratefully accepting the first child that the agency offered them.'

Other excerpts from adoptees' letters show how different they felt from other children or embarrassed by their adoptive status. In many, this is because of their parents' overprotectiveness towards them, based on their own difficulties in having a child, and the fear of having their happiness taken away again. This may touch many chords in the children whose parents had babies as a result of new fertility treatments in later years.

The 'chosen' child story is not, of course, reserved for adoptees. IVF or AID children, too, may be made to feel somehow different, in this way. An antenatal teacher found this idea of the 'special' child very irritating and potentially very problematic:

'One of the mothers at a recent class announced at the beginning that hers was a "very special" baby. I said I was sure every couple here thought their baby was special, but she explained that this baby was the result of years of infertility treatment and three attempts at IVF. Throughout the classes it became clear that her attitude to the birth was very different because of her baby's "specialness". She was quite happy to have a Caesarian or anything the doctors ordered if this was deemed best for her child. Again, this wasn't really any different from the attitude of any of the other mothers. It was just that she had unquestioningly put herself in the hands of "experts" who she felt had achieved her pregnancy for her.

'The baby was born a little premature and was in special care for a few days, but was soon home and a healthy thriving baby. I saw the mother on and off over the next year or two and despite the child's obvious health and robustness she hadn't shaken free of the label of the "special baby". This worried me as I am sure it will cause problems for the child as she gets older.'

Many parents who have had babies only after a long struggle – especially if they only have one child – incline towards over-protecting them. This can cause considerable problems for the children when they reach adolescence and need to separate from their parents. The typical adolescent feels the need to separate from his parents, because only then can he achieve adulthood and the independence to make his own relationships, but at the same time he feels sadness and loneliness in breaking this bond. Hence the adolescent's see-sawing between displays of independence and then demands for attention and affection.

If the parents are secure, they can 'let go' of their adolescents realising that in time a new, more adult bond will be established between them. For the parents of a 'special baby', however, the thought of losing their child is too threatening, reminding them of the long period of pain and loss they experienced while they were infertile and had no child. If the parents send out strong messages that they do not want the child to leave, the child will suffer considerable stress and either feel unable to make the break, remaining emotionally dependent on the parents and perhaps later being unable to form new relationships, or will have to rebel with a vengeance to break free. Whatever the outcome, it is not likely to be good for either parents or children.

STORMY ADOLESCENCES

There is evidence that many adopted children do have particularly stormy adolescences. Many 'act out' their conflicts by
behaving badly, sometimes testing their adoptive parents
love for them by 'running away' to see if their adoptive parents
will abandon them as their birth parents did, or perhaps by
exploring fantasies of the 'bad blood' inherited from the
birth mother or father. If an adolescent girl knows that she
was conceived by a young woman outside of marriage, she
may fantasise that the same thing will happen to her.
Often, adoptive parents will share the same fear and be
particularly concerned about their daughter becoming sexually
active.

Some adopted children do get involved in early sexual
relationships because of this or because they feel a need to get
close to someone, often finding it difficult to form ordinary
relationships with boy- or girl-friends because of a fear of rejection. Some adoptive children actually become pregnant in
order to have a blood relative for the first time. By keeping the
child, the adopted girl can overcome her feelings of
abandonment by her own natural mother by identifying with
the child. Having a baby may also be a way of getting back at
an unsympathetic adoptive mother.

Obviously these are extreme cases and most adopted
children will grow up without such intense problems. But the
fact that these problems can, and do, exist among adopted
children, shows that there may be a need for infertile couples
to be counselled long after they have actually achieved their
'special baby'. They, and their children, may need additional help in overcoming the usual problems of growing
up, and at least be aware of where potential difficulties
exist.

Certainly these cases highlight the adopted child's need for
more information and help in overcoming potential difficulties.
This is now recognised by most professionals concerned with
adoption. They stress the importance of parents working out a
history which shows the child the truth about his origins in a
way he can understand and accept, developing it as he grows in

understanding, and always presenting as positive an image of the child's original parents as possible.

Not giving information is to deny the child not only the truth about himself but also the means to overcome any problems and confusions he might have. It is likely that most adopted children sense, fear or discover the truth about themselves even if their parents conceal it from them, and this could be even more damaging.

SECRECY

The issue of secrecy in adoption and in assisted reproduction techniques such as AID cannot be separated out from other issues concerning the parents', children's and society's feelings. In the past, adoptions were usually considered best kept a secret from the child and from all but the closest relatives who couldn't help knowing about the adoption. This secrecy was considered better for the child, who wouldn't be made to feel insecure, and for the parents, who wouldn't have to be seen as 'inadequate' by society at large.

However, as we have already seen, secrecy gives rise to many problems. A tremendous amount of mental energy has to go into keeping the secret over many years and, as happens with these things, it is liable to burst out at some moment of pressure or crisis, for example on the death of a parent or during a teenage struggle. Adopted children often feel bitter at being told this all-important information so late in the day:

'It was my grandmother who told me, the day after my father died. "He wasn't really your father", she said, "Your parents couldn't have children of their own, you know, you were adopted". Immediately everything fell into place. The fact that my brother and I looked so different (and not very like our parents either). The hesitation and evasion my mother had showed when I tried to talk to her about what childbirth really felt like. A half-remembered conversation when I was small that my mother had with a friend in the kitchen which I had never understood. But the thing that hurt me most was that my grandmother said, "he wasn't really your father". I'm sure that's what my father believed, and I would have done anything, anything to have had the chance to have told him before he died, "You really are my father. You brought me up and I love you". I shall never forgive them for not telling me before it was too late.'

Other adopted children recall being given the stunning information, 'You've turned out just like your real mother!' in the midst of a row, or being told they were adopted at a time when they were feeling at their most insecure. Holding this secret also gives the parents a power over their children which must be unhealthy for the relationship, as many adopted children sense.

WHEN RELATIVES ARE TRACED

It is difficult to understand the controversy over adopted children or adults having access to information about their origins or even tracing their birth parents without realising the extent of the deception to which the adopted child is subjected. When a child is adopted, he or she is given a new birth certificate. This contains the place and date of birth and other details, but replaces the names of the birth parents with the adopting parents and the child's birth name with the name the parents choose to give him or her.

As one adopted person said. 'It is incredible, when you think that what you are given is an officially-sanctioned forgery of a birth certificate. When I finally saw a copy of my original birth certificate, with the name I had first been given and my birth parents' names the extent to which society deceives us adoptees truly hit home.'

In this context, it is interesting to note that since the law was changed under the Children Act 1975 to enable all adopted people over the age of 18 to have access to their original birth records, the great majority of adopted people have not taken up this opening. Similar legislation has now been passed in

Australia, other Commonwealth countries and in some USA states.

Of those adopted people who *do* seek access to their birth records, the majority seek information about their mother and the most frequent questions seem to be, not just ones of fact such as appearance or medical history, which might have consequences for the adopted person and their children, but questions as to why the mother couldn't keep the child, whether the mother still thinks about the child, and if there are other children, siblings or half-siblings for the adopted child. Adopted children sometimes admit to looking in crowds for blood relations or to fears of unknowingly committing incest.

Recent research by Pam Hodgkins, detailed in a report entitled *Adopted adults: an evaluation of their relationships with their families*, was based on questionnaires completed by 181 adoptees who had attempted to trace their birth families. More than three-quarters described their relationship with their adoptive parents when they were a child as average or better, and over half as good. Problems were more common in the teenage years but only a third thought these problems were related to being adopted. Almost three-quarters felt their adult relationship with their parents was average or better.

When describing whether their relationship had changed since tracing the birth parents, two-thirds felt it made no difference, 28 noted improvements while only 16 felt there was a deterioration.

Most research has tended to conclude that it is rare for adoptees to form meaningful relationships with birth parents or families. However, Pam Hodgkins' survey shows that more than three-quarters of adoptees described their relationships with birth parents in positive terms and considered their birth relative to be a friend or used a closer term to describe the relationship. Only three people said that tracing their birth family was a bad decision and seven that it was not worthwhile. Nearly two-thirds of adoptees said they were accepted as a family member by all or most of the birth families or were generally welcomed. Only 20 found the birth relatives indifferent or hostile.

Obviously if an adopted child decides to trace his or her birth parents, the adoptive parents may feel it is a threat – that they will lose their relationship with the child. To some people the idea of their child finding another mother is as threatening as their husband finding another wife or sexual partner.

Adopted children who seek out their parents may therefore find themselves keeping on two separate relationships with their two sets of parents, which can be confusing. 'I just didn't dare tell my mother I was tracing my birth mother, I think she would have been very shocked and hurt. At first I intended just to see if I could trace her, but it was astonishingly easy. I then asked for a meeting, expecting she would say no, but when I met up with her, she was delighted to see me and we got on really well, talked for hours about our lives and so on. I thought that would be it, so I didn't tell my mother, but bit by bit I got more involved and saw more of her, was introduced to my half brothers and sisters, and so on. I can see that it's just how men get involved in an affair and don't manage to tell their wives. The longer it went on, the harder it was to tell my mother that I'd found Sue, my birth mother, and liked her a lot.

'I love my mother and am grateful for everything she's done to bring me up, and I care about her very much. But Sue is very special and I feel she knows me in some curious way that my mother doesn't. There – you see – I still call my mother my mother, to me that's what she is. But I don't feel now I have discovered her that I can stop seeing Sue.'

Some adopted children do find a curious sense of affinity with their blood relations when they meet. And many find the experience of having their own children extraordinary: 'When he was born, I just couldn't believe it. He was my flesh and blood, the first person I had ever seen who was related to me and – astonishingly enough – who looked like me. It reawoke in me my desire to know who my original mother was, and why she had given me away. Because as soon as I saw my child I realised that nothing, nothing would have made me part from him.' (See also *Giving up a baby*, later in this chapter.)

Incest

Sometimes children who seek out their natural parent are reunited with brothers and sisters, too. In some ways such meetings are easier to undertake, as there are no underlying feelings of guilt or resentment, as neither 'gave away' the other, but relationships between separately reared siblings are hard to place in a socially acceptable context. Incestuous feelings may arise. For example, in Britain, counsellors working for NORCAP have become involved in counselling several such cases, which they believe may be the 'tip of an iceberg'. While some reunited siblings say they have nothing in common, many feel very close, and occasionally because of these feelings brothers and sisters reunited in adulthood 'fall in love' with one another.

A well-reported case was that of British couple Terri Bingham and her brother Kim Stalker, separately adopted as children, who were convicted in May 1987 of living together as man and wife, despite being brother and sister by blood. Terri accidentally conceived a child and despite warnings that the child was bound to be born handicapped, she is a normal healthy girl. The couple were told they could only live under the same roof if they had separate bedrooms and lived as brother and sister. Clearly it is impossible to police such a 'crime' and it seems unduly harsh to attempt to intervene in such a relationship.

Psychologists anticipate the risk of this sort of relationship developing; they believe that people 'fall in love' when they recognise similarities in their partner. Often this comes from their family set-up, though it may have to do with inherited personality factors too. The saying 'opposites attract' is simply not true according to these theories. We fall in love with those who are psychologically closest to ourselves and with whom we therefore have, or seem to have, a deep understanding.

If this is the case, does it make the fear of incest voiced by children conceived through AID a real one? Probably not, because the likelihood of AID children meeting is very small – it has been estimated that less than one such marriage would occur every 20 years (see page 78).

However, the fact that these children *might* meet and might find a greater than usual attraction to one another is sufficient reason for ensuring that children born through egg, sperm or embryo donation can check out information about their birth parents. This would at least enable them to discover whether a partner also conceived through donation came from one of the same parent.

STEPFAMILIES

Stepfamilies provide a particularly interesting insight into the possible problems faced by the offspring of sperm or egg donation and surrogate motherhood. In myth and fairy tale, the stepmother is always presented as a wicked usurper, resentful of her stepdaughter's beauty or stepson's prowess who does her best to bring about their downfall, often so that her own children can be elevated in their place.

Psychoanalysts tell us that the fairy godmother and the stepmother really represent the good and bad aspects of the child's mother. Since a small child is totally dependent, he has to believe his mother is perfect and loving. When she acts in an angry, hostile or uncaring way he therefore deals with this by thinking that this is someone else – the stepmother – instead.

Later the child becomes able to fuse these two figures and see that his mother is both good and bad. However, the stories ring uncomfortably true for many children who have been brought up by stepmothers. Why do stepmothers have such a hard time with their stepchildren, and will women bringing up a surrogate mother's child feel the same kinds of conflicts and jealousies?

The myth of the wicked stepmother

Many stepmothers are baffled when they find themselves unwittingly becoming a 'wicked stepmother'. Peggy had a daughter of her own when she married a widower with a two-year-old girl, Laura. The child was only one when her mother had died, so Peggy became the only mother she could remember. Later, Peggy and her husband had another child, Flora, and the three children grew up together as sisters.

Peggy started off with a strong desire to love and care for this 'little motherless child'. But Laura, who had obviously been affected by her mother's death and then being cared for by a series of nannies, initially did not respond to her. Peggy experienced increasing problems in dealing with her stepdaughter. First of all, she found the child reminded her forcefully of her husband's ex-wife, who she knew through photographs, and she found this very disturbing. Secondly, the child was very insecure and tried so hard to please that Peggy found herself irritated by Laura being the 'good girl' while her two other daughters were their normal, noisy selves. Laura also played up to her father's guilt and protectiveness towards her and this angered Peggy too. Peggy never felt close enough to Laura to feel comfortable about punishing her or sharing in the physical intimacies which came so naturally to her with her other children.

As time went by, Peggy and Laura came to dislike and mistrust one another more and more, and rivalries and jealousies sprang up between the three sisters too. Peggy became increasingly confused as she found herself more and more resentful of the unhappiness in the family. Because she could not understand why it had happened, she blamed the personality of her stepdaughter as chiefly responsible.

This kind of story is not uncommon. Many of the problems stepmothers face come from the fact that a stepchild reminds them of their predecessor and the physical bond between child and father. This makes it hard for them to feel other than jealous and resentful of the child. Stepmothers are often obliged to care for another woman's child without having time to get to know them well and without the experience of pregnancy, birth and the knowledge that the child is theirs to break down the natural barriers that we have with other people. Perhaps most important, most stepmothers did not choose this role; they had to accept the child in order to have a relationship with the father. A situation which is foisted on you rather than chosen is far more likely to lead to resentment and other problems.

Are mothers of children born to surrogates likely to feel the same? One wonders. Photographs of Kim Cotton and her baby showed that her baby bore a strong resemblance to this striking woman, as did the children of her marriage. Somewhere a mother is bringing up this child knowing that she looks like her natural mother, who, by campaigning in support of surrogate motherhood has become a semi-public figure. What will the child's mother feel about this and how will she deal with her feelings?

Stepfathers – some sobering facts

The role of the stepfather is, if anything, more difficult to handle than that of the stepmother. Many cases of child abuse – including those which received great publicity such as that of Jasmine Beckford and Maria Colwell – were the result of battering or torture by a stepfather. Again, a stepfather might feel the same jealousies of the child's father and the sexual relationship between his present wife and her former husband. But because of cultural attitudes, in a man these might take on a more violent form.

Stepfathers, too, possibly face difficulties in trying to discipline a child with whom they do not have an intimate relationship and to whom they might have taken on the paternal role soon after their first meeting. As one stepfather, now happy with his new family, said, 'It's very hard to cope with them when every time I tell them what to do they turn around and say, "You can't say that, you're not my father".'

When stepfamily relationships go wrong, they often do so with a vengeance. In our society, as in most, sexual relationships between father and daughter, mother and son, are strongly prohibited. However, this taboo is not clear-cut between biologically unrelated step-parents and children. Perhaps because of this lack of taboo, many cases of incest or child sexual abuse involve stepfathers.

Those who have studied and written about stepfamilies have come to the firm conclusion that being a step-parent and a parent are two very different things, even if the child's original mother or father has died or lost all contact and the step-parent is taking on the full parental responsibilities. They recommend that step-parents do not expect too much of their relationship with the child.

The fathers of AID children may find themselves to some extent in the same position as the stepfather. Of course, there are differences, too. The children will never have known any other father with AID, while those who now live with a stepfather may know their natural father. Also, the stepfather may have other children of his own.

However, some infertile men whose children were conceived through AID do have fantasies about the donor in much the same way as a stepfather might have fantasies about his step-child's natural father. Although there was never a physical relationship between the donor and the wife or partner of the AID father, a symbolic union has taken place which may cause conscious or unconscious jealousies.

As one AID father said, 'I used to wonder who he (the donor) was. I'd look at my son and try to piece together what his father would be like from the child's features which didn't seem to come from his mother. Because the donor was fertile and I wasn't, I thought he was somehow better than me. I imagined him as a cocky young man always ready for sex. I used to wonder if I'd recognise him if I bumped into him in a supermarket.'

Teenagers and step-parents

Step-parents seem to face particular problems when their step-children become teenagers; will the same apply to parents of children born of AID or through surrogate mothers? The teenage years are difficult for many parents because their children take up different viewpoints, challenge their parent's attitudes, want to do things their way and may find it hard to compromise. They may also express hostility or dislike of their parents' way of life or aspects of their personalities. Many parents have problems coping with this process of rejection which is necessary if the teenagers are ever to move away from the parental home and become adults in their own right.

If the parents are insecure about their relation to the child, this can cause extra pain to them, as they may feel they are being rejected not because they are a parent, but because they are not enough of a parent – not a genetic as well as social parent. They may feel the child is 'turning on them' because of this or that the parts of the child's personality inherited from the donor or surrogate are coming to the fore. Parents of adopted children also feel these fears.

Unlike the studies of children in adoptive families, what studies there are of how children fare in step-families do not give such a reassuring picture of the children's development. Considering the scale of divorce and remarriage, it is rather surprising that so little material on step-families exists. One estimate is that one in five children born in Britain in 1980 will experience parental divorce before they are 16.

Research shows that children with stepfathers are much more likely than those in unbroken families to have poor relationships with their fathers. The same applies to children with stepmothers, and in both cases relationships are likely to be worse if the original family was broken by divorce than if a parent died. The children do not seem to have a poorer view of their remarried natural parent or have more conflict with siblings.

Children with stepfathers seem to have lower aspirations and want to leave school earlier, especially boys; this is not true of children with stepmothers. Parents with step-children are more likely to see their sons and daughters as showing problem behaviour than those in unbroken homes.

Recent research has shown that the effect of divorce on a family may be long-lasting, and it may be true that some of the problems faced by children in step-families results from the trauma of divorce and perhaps from continuing ill-feeling between the separated spouses over access and the children generally. Divorced fathers are more likely to lose touch with their children entirely following divorce. It may be that boys experience more difficulties with stepfathers because the stepfather does not provide the interest, support and encouragement that the natural father would have provided.

Whatever the complete picture is, the problems faced by stepchildren must be considered when looking at how the children born of donated eggs, embryos and sperm or of surrogate mothers will feel. The step-family seems an unenviable set-up. Are the families we are creating through egg, sperm and embryo donation likely to become like modern step-families?

Some important differences

While the similarities between such families and step-families might indicate potential problems, it is important to be aware also of the considerable differences. The stepchild was never intended for life in a step-family; the step-parent never planned to take him on. However, people who are prepared to have a child with another biological parent want this child enormously. Also, usually they do not know the donor, and neither does the child, so that even after being told of his or her existence, the donor cannot take on the role of the child's 'real' parent in the way that a step-parent does. The donor is far less of a threat and cannot interfere in the way that an existing ex-wife or husband can.

This is one reason why many doctors and counsellors think an unknown donor is better for parents and child than a known donor who might later try to influence or interfere in the relationships within the new family.

People who have had a child through a surrogate mother may find themselves closer to the situation of a step-parent. In many surrogate cases, the surrogate mother and the mother-to-be are in contact throughout the pregnancy so that the mother-to-be can share in the experience of watching her baby grow and develop, and feel reassured. However, these experiences may mean that when the baby is handed over, the surrogate mother remains an important figure whose influence and memory linger on. After the birth most ties are broken perhaps because all parties find contact a strain.

Because surrogate motherhood is outside the law, there is always the possibility that the surrogate mother might decide to keep the child or even claim that she wants the child back after he or she has been handed over. Because of this, the surrogate mother is a potential threat to the future happiness of the couple involved and so can be feared or hated in the same way that an ex-spouse might be.

Where there is a dispute over the future of the child and, as in America, the child been awarded to the commissioning couple with the surrogate mother granted access, the surrogate mother could fit the same role as the ex-wife in a step-family.

There are similarities here to adoption, too. When a couple are to adopt a baby, the natural mother has the right to change her mind up until the time when the adoption is actually heard, which can take some time. Because of this, couples might fear the natural mother and see her as a possible wrecker of their happiness. If couples develop such feelings about a natural mother, a surrogate mother or an ex-spouse, parent of their stepchild, it is clearly very difficult for them to do what they are supposed to; provide a positive image of the child's natural or biological parent so that the child does not feel that his original parent, and thus himself, is 'bad'.

Giving up a baby

Certainly there is a very real risk of the natural mother wishing to have her child returned to her – or at least some contact, however tenuous. Studies of women who relinquished their babies for adoption show how painful, and often lastingly so, the experience can be. One national study in Australia of 213 women who had given up a first child for adoption when young and single showed that the effects on the mother were extremely negative and long-lasting. Half the women reported an increasing sense of loss over periods of up to 30 years.

Many of these women felt that the sense of loss could in fact have been eased by having some information about the fate of their offspring, but for most this was not available either from the agencies through whom they had given up their children or other sources. The individual stories told by some of these mothers are heart-rending. One, bowing to social pressure, gave up her first-born baby daughter after birth, tears falling on the form consenting to the adoption as she signed it. Later she married the father of the baby and had two sons, but could never get the thought of her lost daughter from her mind, scanning the faces of children of about her age in the hope that she might recognise her daughter. Another mother recalls leaving her baby on the table at the adoption agency and walking out, the sound of the baby's screams filling her ears, a sound which she has never been able to forget.

In the study written up in *The Adoption Triangle*, the authors interviewed 38 birth parents in depth, 36 mothers and 2 fathers. All the babies were adopted in the first six months, three-quarters in the first week. Most babies were given up because the parents were unmarried, too young and unprepared for parenthood.

Though the majority of these parents had given up their babies 10 to 33 years ago, 50 per cent said they still experienced feelings of loss, pain and mourning; 53 per cent would like the child to know that they cared about him or her; 82 per cent wondered what the child looked like, how he or she was growing up and whether he was well-cared for. Also, 82 per cent said they would like to be reunited with the child when he or she reached adulthood, though 87 per cent said they did not want to hurt the adoptive parents. A staggering 95 per cent said that they would like to update the information about themselves in their records, many to show that they had now made a success of their life and that they were not people to be ashamed of.

Other studies on adoption and letters from birth parents show that most relinquishing mothers fear that their child will never forgive them for abandoning him or her, and want to have the opportunity to show that they do care, and that they did what they did for love of the child and to give him or her a better life. Because of this continued interest felt by birth parents for their child, the lack of any information given to the relinquishing mothers by the agencies seems rather hard. One birth mother wrote repeatedly to the adoption agency, begging simply to be told if the child was alive and well, only to be told that all records had been lost.

Nowadays, adoption agencies are likely to be more open, giving information to the natural mother about the adoptive parents and sometimes allowing access to the child if all parties are agreeable. However, even if a mother believes that adoption was the best thing she could do for her child at that time, when circumstances change in her life she may then wish to have the child back or wish she had acted otherwise, something which will be a continuous source of pain to her and which is not possible if she has had an abortion. Every adoptive mother probably fears that one day a distraught birth mother will appear wanting her child back, and it is understandable that most want to be protected from this possibility. It is also a possibility, as we have already seen, that this will occur in cases of surrogate motherhood.

SUMMING UP

There are clearly no easy answers to the questions raised in this chapter. The suggestion that adopted children, and children born through artificial insemination by donor, egg and embryo donation and surrogate motherhood might be allowed to know how they were conceived and to have information about their parents or even be enabled to trace them, clearly makes many uncomfortable. 'I wouldn't even consider AID if my child would be told about it', said one potential father. One AID counsellor was even quoted as saying that if children were to be given the identity of the donor, she would 'burn all the records' in her clinic.

This is reminiscent of the feelings displayed by many adoptive parents at the time that adopted children were given the right of access to their original birth records, that 'We adopted the children so they would be ours, not so that we could act as babysitters till a reunion with the birth parents came about.'

However, most adoptive parents now realise that they adopted to have a chance to parent, not to 'own' their child, and that the child has a right to know its background. Those who have used and will use the new reproductive technologies will do best to learn by their experience. If society is to press ahead with these treatments this right needs to be enforced so that the children conceived of this 'brave new world' can voice their views in openness and honesty. Only then will we be able to judge how successful these new treatments for infertility have been, and be assured that the children born of them will not be harmed.

Further Reading List

Test-tube Women by R. Arditti etc, Pandora Press, 1984

The Myth of Motherhood by Elizabeth Badinter, Souvenir Press, 1982

Baby Cotton – For Love and Money by Kim Cotton and Denise Winn, Dorling Kindersley, 1985

Babymaking by Susan Downie, Bodley Head, 1988

The Experience of Infertility by Naomi Pfeffer and Anne Woollett, Virago, 1983

Coping with Childlessness by Diane and Peter Houghton, Unwin, 1987

Taking Chances: Abortion and the Decision Not to Contracept by Kristen Luker, University of California Press, 1976

The Gift of a Child by Elizabeth and Robert Snowden, Allen & Unwin, 1984

The Artificial Family by R. Snowden and G. D. Mitchell, Allen & Unwin, 1981

Surrogate Mother: One Woman's Story by Kirsty Stevens and Emma Dally, Century, 1985

Adoption Triangle by Arthur Sorosky et al, Doubleday, 1978

Adoption: A Second Chance by Barbara Tizard, Open Books, 1977

Infertility: A Sympathetic Approach by Robert Winston, Macdonald Optima, 1987

Useful Addresses

Be My Parent
c/o *BAAF* (address below)
Tel: 01 – 407 9763

Book produced by BAAF containing two hundred photographs
and descriptions of children with special needs looking for
families. Telephone for information on where the nearest book
can be seen.

British Agencies for Adoption and Fostering (BAAF)
11 Southwark Street
London SE1 1RQ
Tel: 01 – 407 8800

Promotes good standards of practice in adoption and fostering
and aims to increase public understanding of the social, legal,
medical and psychological issues involved in adoption. BAAF
provides an advisory service and publishes the booklet 'Adopting a Child' each year giving up-to-date information for
would-be adopters.

British Pregnancy Advisory Service
Austy Manor,
Wooten Wawen
Solihull
West Midlands
Tel: 05642 – 3225

BPAS provides counselling and infertility services for couples who find difficulty in obtaining the help they need through the National Health Service. They provide a full infertility investigation, AIH and AID, vasectomy and sterilization reversals, laparoscopy and tubal repair if necessary. A leaflet with more details and fees is available on request.

Child
'Farthings'
Pawlett
Near Bridgwater
Somerset
Tel: 0278 – 683595

Provides information for those who are not able to conceive. A newsletter and fact sheets are available. A 24-hour information service is available on the above number.

Family Planning Association
27 – 35 Mortimer Street
London W1N 7RJ
Tel: 01 – 636 7866

As well as providing information on contraception and sexuality, the FPA will give advice and information on infertility.

The Miscarriage Association
PO Box 24
Ossett
West Yorkshire WF5 9XG
Tel: 0924 – 830515

Provides support, help and information for women and their families who have had, or are having, a miscarriage. It produces leaflets, pamphlets and a newsletter and can also refer people to local groups.

Parent to Parent Information on Adoptive Services (PPIAS)
Lower Boddington
Daventry
Northamptonshire NN11 6YB
Tel: 0327 – 60295

Helps potential adopters by passing on information about how and where to apply for children, especially those with special needs, and also from overseas. Local groups also give support to members who have adopted or are in the process of doing so.

Progress
27 – 35 Mortimer Street
London W1N 7RJ
Tel: 01 – 580 9360

Campaign supporting research on embryos.

National Association for the Childless
318 Summer Lane
Birmingham B19 3RL
Tel: 021 – 359 4887

Provides advice, information and support to childless couples – both counselling for people with infertility problems and helping the childless to find a fulfilled life-style. Members can be referred to local contacts, many of whom run self-help groups. A newsletter and fact sheets on childlessness are available.

National Childbirth Trust
9 Queensborough Terrace
Bayswater
London W2 3TB
Tel: 01 – 221 3833

As well as promoting education for parenthood and supporting choice in childbirth, NCT's post-natal support group will provide information and support for parents who have lost a baby.

National Association for Counselling Adoptees and their Parents (NORCAP)
3 New High Street
Headington
Oxford OX3 7AJ
Tel: 0865 – 750554

Provides support to adult adopted people and both their adoptive and birth parents. Helps adult adopted people who are trying to get in touch with their birth parents and has a register of both adoptees and birth relatives seeking to make contact.

National Stepfamily Association
329 Mills Road
Cambridge CB2 2QT
Tel: 0223 – 246861
Information and support for step-parents and children.

Relate (National Marriage Guidance Council)
Herbert Gray College
Little Church Street
Rugby, Warwickshire CV21 3AP
Tel: Rugby 0788 – 73241
Provides confidential counselling for couples with marriage or relationship problems, whatever the cause.

Stepfamily
Maris House
Maris Lane
Trumpington
Cambridge CB2 2LB
Tel: 0223 – 841306

The Stillbirth and Neonatal Death Society (SANDS)
Argyle House
29 – 31 Euston Road
London NW1 2SD
Tel: 01 – 436 5881
Offers information and support for parents who have been bereaved through a national network of parents.

Voluntary Licensing Authority
20 Park Crescent
London W1N 4AL
Tel: 01 – 636 5422
Will provide a list of approved IVF clinics.

Women's Reproductive Rights Information Centre
Women's Aid Centre
51 Chalcot Road
London NW1
Tel: 01 – 586 0104
Information concerning infertility, family planning and abortion.

Index